Seven STEPS TO CHIROPRACTIC SUCCESS

A Comprehensive Guide for the Chiropractic Professional

F. Michael Anderson, D.C. • Micheil Hanczaryk, D.C.
William M. Harris, D.C. • David J. Kats, D.C.
Lloyd E. Latch, D.C. • David S. Singer, D.C.
John T. Whitney, D.C.

Introduction by David C. Lindsey, D.C.

d'Carlin Publishing
P.O. Box 534
Carlsbad, CA 92008

For information address d'Carlin Publishing, P.O. Box 534, Carlsbad, CA 92008, (619) 729-7758.

Editorial Supervision by David C. Lindsey, D.C.
Typesetting by Headline Advertising, Encinitas, CA

ISBN: 0-939342-03-0

Printed in the U.S.A.

Acknowledgement

The co-authors wish to acknowledge the contributions made to the chiropractic profession by all the pioneers and those who have raised the profession to its present state of recognition.

CONTENTS

INTRODUCTION
A New Perspective

Recently I asked a chiropractic college educator why students didn't receive some help in learning the business side of the profession.

"We have our hands full teaching the fundamentals required to pass the State Board . . . While we appreciate the need for this knowledge, it's the responsibility of the individual to get this information and training from another source, a business school or through post-graduate seminars."

No doubt the identical explanation holds true for graduates of all professions, law, engineering, architecture, etc. This could be why every solicitation I receive for expanding one's career by attending a "management" course includes testimonials from highly placed individuals in every profession, as well as endorsements from Fortune 500 executives.

And, I suppose, the life of "How to Win Friends and Influence People" is infinite . . . because individuals from all walks of life can benefit from additional help to reach the top of the heap.

So, what's wrong with wanting to be better than you are?

It's the American way, ask any athlete or fan why the coach takes the heat during a losing season . . . isn't it because winning is better?

Some athletic teams gain nicknames from their winning attitude, but so do the losers. And, conversely, the Mets got some of their greatest support during their sorriest streak of losing. We can love a loser sometimes, but not often.

What does "management counseling" have to do with athletics? Just this, through a solution-seeking process, a consult can retrain each office member to function like a sports team, where player, trainer and coach function as a single unit. Now, the doctor, CA and office manager pursue a common goal, greater patient benefits . . . the environment for success.

If we agree on this, why should there exist an aura of skepticism regarding "Chiropractic Management Consultants?" Just because a professional is a highly individualized person is no reason to exclude the services of those who could contribute to your success in problem areas of communication, staff and finances.

The triangle of total health: Nutrition, Structural Balance, and Emotional Well-being has its counterpart in the chiropractic office:

1) Communication
2) A goal-oriented staff
3) Financial strength

The doctor demonstrates his skill through his adjustment techniques, a powerful line of communication to patients. The staff must be supportive, cooperative and dedicated to the goals of the office, which are in reality established by the needs of patients. Without financial stability, the whole structure exists temporarily on shaky grounds.

What can the services of a management consultant do to bring all three needs of a successful practice into focus?

This is the problem that management people solve, uncovering the blocks to success. Admittedly, this is a sensitive undertaking, but it's a far better decision than allowing the deterioration of a correctable condition to reach a terminal stage.

Each of the co-authors of *Seven Steps to Chiropractic*

Success have proven their ability to fashion a successful practice. . .either through trial-and-error or intensive years of observation and training. Now they want to make other doctors equally successful and healthy.

Of course, there's no free lunch. . .your patients don't get one from you. Education is expensive at whatever level, college or post-college. But, nothing is more expensive than under-exploiting your full potential to reach goals which put you in command, on top of your career.

You deserve consideration equal to what you provide your patients. . .total health in every area of daily life.

You'll find several recipes for success within the pages of this book. Any one of them can return your investment in *Seven Steps to Chiropractic Success.*

You're ready to start your journey up the ladder.

David C. Lindsey, D.C.

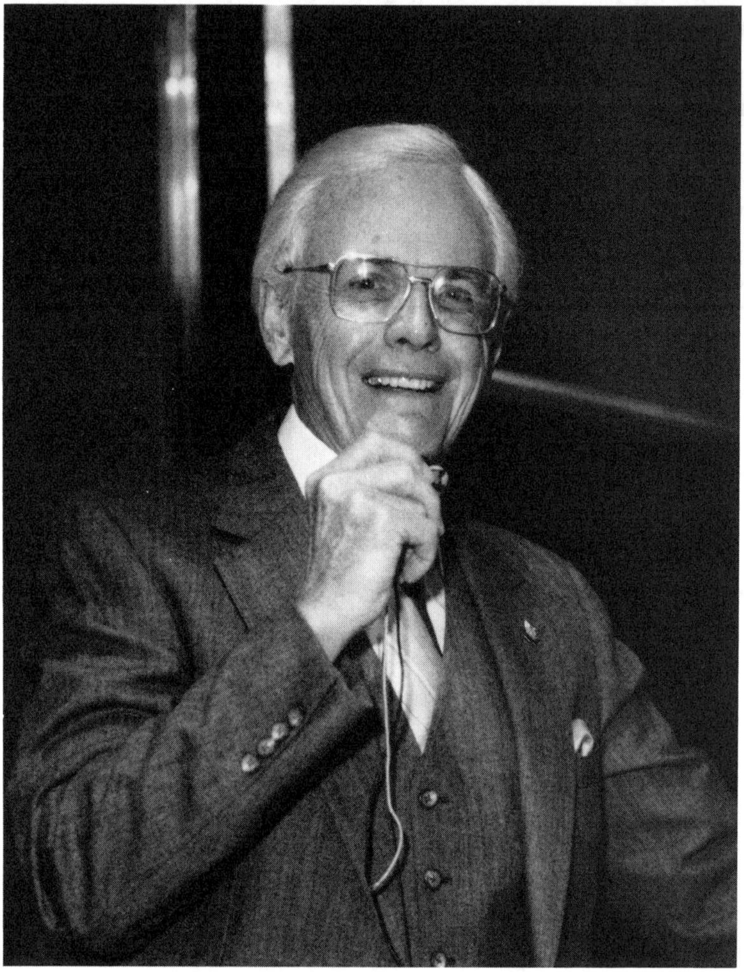

William M. Harris, D.C.

WILLIAM M. HARRIS, D.C.
PRACTICE CONSULTANTS

Dr. William M. Harris has personally and individually taught more successful chiropractors than any other. He has the unique talent as a teacher to give you and your staff a higher self-worth, ideas to up your income, and inspirational motivation to enable you to rise to your fullest and highest potential.

In 1973, Dr. Harris opened a new quarter-million dollar clinic for "in-patient" and "out-patient" care . . . the first in Georgia.

Dr. Harris began PRACTICE CONSULTANTS in 1974. Chiropractors are taught via lecture, T.V. demonstrations, individual conferences, etc., by the highly trained PRACTICE CONSULTANTS staff.

Success is a science. Let PRACTICE CONSULTANTS teach you the science of success.

You too can retire by applying PRACTICE CONSULTANTS' principles of success.

PRACTICE CONSULTANTS
526 Broad Avenue, Albany, Georgia 31702
(912) 888-1927

NOTES / GOALS:

CHAPTER 1
The Attitude of Success
William M. Harris, D.C.

In the late fifties, I was asked to conduct a week's seminar in "practice and business management" to every graduating class at Palmer College. (This was during the lifetime of Dr. B.J. Palmer.)

In one particular graduating class, I picked out two students and predicted that they both would be outstanding achievers in their chosen profession. Since they were both from the South, I kept in touch and noted their progress.

Dr. Frank (not his true name but the story nevertheless is real) received help from his family in opening an office. From the very beginning he did exceptionally well. Success came easy for him. He married and continued to prosper. Soon he bought a new home. His wife became pregnant and he continued to prosper. It seemed that backsets and failures eluded him. After a time, for a number of reasons, he and his wife divorced.

Being a successful doctor, with his new-found freedom

and a good-looking car, Dr. Frank found it easy to date whomever he asked. Soon his concentration began to drift from his chief talent as a doctor and he became preoccupied with "womanizing." During this time he began to live beyond his income, but he found it easy to borrow to cover the deficit.

In due time, he married again. He had to reestablish a new home and furnishings for his new wife and begin his second family. He did not worry because he found it easy to borrow from the bank. In the meantime, he was gradually getting into a state of losing control of financial reality and financial responsibility. When he would have several poor months of practice income and the bank notes became due, he began to escape, temporarily, from his pressures by drinking.

It was only a matter of time before he lost his nice clinic building. His equipment was sold to meet bank obligations and the last report was that he was not mentally, emotionally or financially able to engage in his talent as a chiropractor.

The next man in the same graduating class (we will call him Dr. Ed) had a very difficult time in borrowing money to open a meager office. He had never been in the world of business before. Because he had more compassion than he had capital reserve, he told his patients, "Don't worry about your bill." That is one piece of advice that patients will always follow!

He literally failed in practice and had to move his office to another town. He learned from his failure and resolved to learn the rudiments of practice management in order to profit from his failure.

In other words, Dr. Ed learned early that failure is a part of the process of ultimately succeeding. Whereas, Dr. Frank had no failures and was not able to cope with failure because his success had come so easily.

Dr. Ed married a very supportive wife and they became a part of the social, civic, and religious aspects of the community. He realized from his first experience to never overextend his obligations and to strive to have extra money in reserve for emergencies. As a result, his progress and income were slower in building than Dr. Frank, but his progress was steady.

Dr. Ed has several different offices in one of the largest cities in the South. He is continuing to expand and has become a highly respected man in his profession as well as in his city.

WHAT MAKES THE DIFFERENCE?

What made the difference in the two men who started out with great potentials? As I review, it would be simply two words - attitude and commitment.

Dr. Ed never lost sight of his primary commitments - servicing his patients and becoming eventually solvent. He learned from his early failure.

Dr. Frank, because he had no failures and success came very easily, learned too late that when you spend your means and let your commitment as a chiropractor become secondary, you are headed for a debtor's spiral. His attitude soured and so did his commitment to his personal responsibilities.

WHERE DO ATTITUDE AND COMMITMENT BEGIN?

When Practice Consultants[1] first began ten years ago, we resolved to find out: What were the key factors that made one person succeed and another person, seemingly with similar talents, fail to make his/her mark, and why there were so many chiropractors who never got beyond "subsistence" income.

Practice Consultants employed a leading psychologist and a well-known psychiatrist. They each were asked, "What makes one person succeed and another ultimately become average or fail?" Both professionals contended that it was to a great degree determined by the person's self-image or self-worth; that between the ages of three and five the self-image and self-worth of an individual were formed. They further stated that, with few exceptions, most individuals kept this image of self, formed at this early age, for the rest of their lives. Figure 1 is a graph illustrating the substance of the psychiatrist's and the psychologist's information.

Are you aware that if, during this crucial period between the ages of three and five, you received positive strokes (strokes mean encouragement and building your faith and confidence) from your parents and close relatives, you had an image embedded in you that you were a worthy person, and that you ultimately succeeded because of this early environment which cultivated a successful outlook on your ability and your future?

Likewise, in the middle of the graph, you will notice

[1]*Foundation for the Advancement of Chiropractic Education — the first management firm in the field of chiropractic to become non-profit and the first in the chiropractic management field to fund a $50,000.00-per-year "chair" in practice and business management at Palmer College. Other chairs will be funded with other colleges as time progresses.*

that people who received very little encouragement and few strokes and were constantly having to adjust their response to the home life and to living to suit the whims of their parents in order to receive love (unless there was a drastic desire or change later in their psyche) became the average people of the world - even though they may have had the capacity to exceed those who ultimately won.

Notice in the right-hand column that the bitter losers

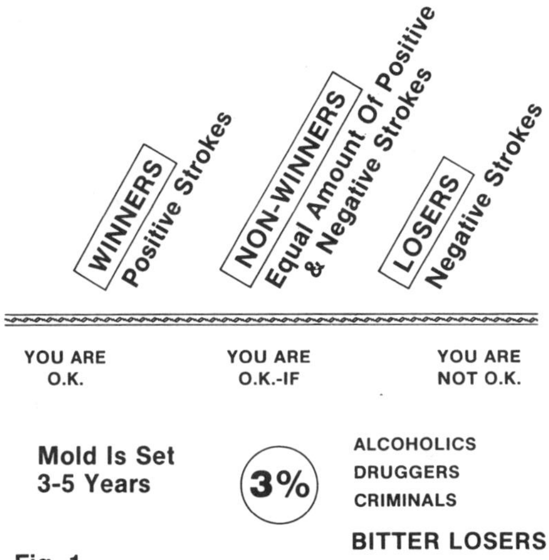

Fig. 1

were the ones who became (unless a drastic change happened in their lives at a later period) problems in the social structure of society.

It all begins with an attitude containing self-worth and a self-image.

Because of my early childhood, I was "programmed" literally to fail and history records that I became a very "successful failure."

In the early incubation period of my life, between three and five years, my mother became ill and was taken from the home, and my father lost his spirit and desire to continue to succeed as he had in the past. Thus I was in an environment of constant sadness and financial strife. There were no words of encouragement that told me I was entitled to achieve the benefits or the blessings of success.

Because of a personal experience with chiropractic, I entered the Palmer College and there I met my future wife, an X-ray technician at the college. For the first time in my life, through her words of encouragement, bitterness began to lessen in my outlook and attitude and I began to be encouraged that I could, in due time, through her faith and belief in me, become a success.

ATTITUDES AND GOALS

My first office was in the basement of a theater building in McDonough, Georgia. The rent was $15.00 per month. Hoping to increase my financial position, I opened a branch office 18 miles away in Jackson, Georgia. Little did I know that my overhead would double but my income would not.

It was during this period of time that my wife and I learned that Napoleon Hill, author of the best-selling book, "Think and Grow Rich," was going to conduct a series of lectures in Atlanta, Georgia, on the principles of success which he had gleaned from personally studying the lives of 500 of America's wealthiest millionaires.

At the encouragement of my wife, we attended these weekly sessions conducted by Mr. Hill and began to apply the principles - which are as immutable as the law of gravity - to our circumstances.

We set our goals to retire at age 35 and we only missed this by one year.

GOALS AND YOUR FUTURE

Napoleon Hill furnished examples of the importance of having concrete, written goals, reading them on a regular basis, and during the reading to visualize yourself in possession of the goals you desire.

He stated the subconscious mind has a tremendous role in a person's ultimate future and success. It was the guiding factor, if fed the right suggestions and food, and would help in its own omnipotent way to bring success to your life. He said, further, that many people questioned the validity of the approach but no one was able to refute the benefits of the approach when it came to results obtained.

When you change your objective mind (the mind you use every day) to decide definitely and specifically on the things and the goals you DESIRE, you have begun the first step in accomplishing or securing what you really want. With persistence, your goals become real.

When you tune in a radio correctly, you get a perfect result, but to do this it is necessary to know something of the radio and its plan of operation. Likewise, you have within you a "mighty power." It is anxious and willing to serve you in a constructive way – a power capable of giving you that which you earnestly DESIRE.

This power of the subconscious mind, described by many authors, is especially well written about by Thomas J. Hudson, Ph.D., LL.D., in his book, "The Law of Psychic Phenomena." Many other learned writers in the field of success use different names, but all agree that it is omnipotent. Therefore, let us call it the "God within you" or "divine intelligence."

Occasionally making a halfhearted wish does not form a perfect connection or communication with your omnipotent power. You must be in earnest, persistent, sincere and truthful in desiring certain things or conditions in the mental, physical or spiritual route.

Your thinking mind (objective mind) will tend to vacillate, therefore, you usually only wish for things. As a result, the capable, wonderful power within you does not function to bring about your wishes because most wishes are simple mental expressions.

If you are in earnest about changing your present circumstances, here is a simple, definite, resultful, concise method with rules, explanations and suggestions which has worked in the lives of countless doctors who have used Practice Consultants' services with outstanding benefit.

At this time, write down the things, the goals and the conditions you really want in your life. Go to the limit of your desires. Rearrange the list daily, adding to or taking from the list, until you have listed the seven most important things that you want to accomplish in your life in the next twelve months. Do not be discouraged on account of changes that you make in the list initially. There will always be changes and additions with accomplishments and increased success.

THREE TESTED RULES OF ACCOMPLISHMENT

1) Think with intensity and feeling in your allowable moments during the day about what you really want. Do this as often as possible. Imagine that you already possess the goal or the ideal condition desired.
2) It is important that you read (preferably aloud) the list of what you want a MINIMUM of three times each day - morning, noon and night.
3) Under no circumstances do you talk to anyone about your plans or goals except to the "great power" (the

"God power" or "divine intelligence") within you which will, in turn, gradually but assuredly unfold to your objective mind the method of accomplishment.

Some of your goals, from practical reasoning, may seem at the moment unattainable. However, write them down on your list in the proper order of their importance to your success.

It is obvious that you cannot acquire faith in the simplicity of this principle at the start, but can you, for example, figure out why a seed placed in fertile soil shoots up in due time a beautiful flower?

By following this simple, specific plan, which has worked in the countless lives of other Practice Consultants' clients and worked in the life of Napoleon Hill, the method of ultimate success will unfold just as mysteriously as a seed planted in soil produces the visible result in the form of a beautiful flower and, in many instances, much faster than you expect.

Faith in the principles develops as you experience your goals being accomplished.

If you want money, write down the amount, be practical and reasonable. If you want to break existing records in your practice, write them down. This procedure may seem foolish at first, but are you aware that you can never realize your desires or successes if you do not positively and in detail reduce to writing what you want and when you want it?

Many people, unfortunately, take more time in planning their vacations than they do in planning the goals for the achievements in their lives.

If you cannot decide on your goals, you are not in earnest. By being definite and reading the list on a consistent daily basis, thinking about these goals being real in your life, and not talking to another single person about them, the results will be surprising to you and sometimes almost unbelievable.

"It's impossible!" "It would have happened anyway." "What is so remarkable?" Many times these are the remarks of the skeptic when the first goal on their list is accomplished. A natural enemy, doubt, will appear. Be cautious not to discredit the principles outlined, which are as immutable as the laws of nature (the law of gravity, for example).

When a goal is accomplished in your list, give thanks to divine intelligence. Give credit to the power within you for the accomplishment. By doing this, you gain assurance, accomplish more and, in time, prove beyond a shadow of a doubt that there is an immutable law which actually works - unfailingly - when you are in tune with it!

The power within and what it does is beyond total human understanding. Do not try to understand it, but accept the accomplishments with thankfulness and strengthened faith. This simple method of obtaining your desires is powerful.

It is suggested that your first list of goals consist of those things with which you are quite familiar, such as possession of material things, an amount of money, and so forth.

Such goals as these are more easily obtained than changing the welfare of others and changing the healing of others. To gain confidence in the simplicity of these immutable laws, accomplish the lesser things first. As these are accomplished, you will seek the higher and more important objectives. Long before you have reached this stage, you will find many of your goals will have been realized and erased from your list.

Be cautious that you do not place on your list things which will ultimately make you miserable or will wreck the happiness of others.

One goal, I feel, should be to help others as you are being helped. Is it not a great reward to those who assist and give unselfishly? It is impossible to be unselfish without gain.

Many people reject chiropractic because of its simplicity. Likewise, you may reject or accept the simplicity of the plan for obtaining goals as herein outlined. The choice is yours.

It is my earnest prayer that you may find faith and assistance in these words on goals. (It is recommended to read this section over and over daily for a minimum of one month to have total comprehension and absorption.) Follow the simplicity of the plan and thereby obtain, as have countless others, the things which are your heart's desire.

It has been my experience that poverty is self-inflicted through choices, feelings and actions. Likewise, riches are self-imposed through definite planning and definite goals written out and persistently pursued until accomplished.

THE CHIROPRACTIC EXPLOSION

Are you aware that chiropractic is undergoing a tremendous growth explosion? There are more students of chiropractic today than there have ever been in the history of chiropractic.

It has been estimated that one out of three graduates will leave the profession at the end of two years because:

1) They have found they are not mentally or emotionally suited to the demands of a professional life or of listening to the complaints of sick patients day in and day out.

2) They have not learned the second phase of becoming a success – the management phase of a professional life.

In this period of history, Dr. Jim Parker has done much to give some broad principles of management to the profession and many have benefited from his seminars.

I was very successful in practice when I learned of Dr. Jim's seminars. I attended his second seminar which was held in Atlanta, Georgia, and have since that time encouraged others to obtain this basic information.

When the graduate leaves school, he/she has learned only one phase of becoming a success, and that is the technical side of becoming adequate in X-ray interpretation, digital palpation, diagnosis, and so forth. There is another phase that is a prerequisite for the successful person, and that is learning the practical business management procedures essential to develop a successful practice. As I see it, there are two ways that this can be accomplished:

1) You can learn through the school of hard knocks, through trial and error, the answers to all practice problems over a period of years.
2) You can obtain the services of a management firm that has a tested track record and years of experience in teaching and coaching on a one-to-one basis. You would be taught all the things necessary to make your practice succeed and, shown through a computer review of your practice, how to "plug the leaks" in your income as well as ways to increase your new patient flow.

LOCATION AND SIZE OF YOUR OFFICE SPACE

According to research by the American Medical Association, it has been estimated that 85% of a doctor's success is determined by his location.

It is far better to have a location on a prominent street and pay slightly more for the space than to have a savings through opening your office on a side street where your sign and your presence are not visible to the masses. It is wise to have your location on a street where the traffic is not going more than 30 miles per hour. On a freeway, your sign is not noticed as quickly because the driving attention is on the road and other cars.

A true example of saving pennies and losing dollars is a friend of mine who, through false economy, bought a lot on a side street because it was more reasonable. In due time, he built a handsome structure. He attended countless seminars to improve his professional skills. Yet in the town where he practices, very few people know of where his location is or the fact that he is in town simply because he is on a little-traveled street. I have often wondered just how successful he would have been, because he is technically proficient, if he had chosen a more desirable location.

For a single practitioner, there should be no less than a minimum of 800 to a maximum of 1,200 square feet. A lesser amount of space will handicap you quickly and will block your growth and expansion.

YOUR LEASE AND ITS IMPORTANCE

You, the citizen, to open a practice and operate it using competent financial and management counsel, recall to me a lesson taught in the favorite story of "The Three Little Pigs."

Two of the pigs, as you recall, upon leaving home put together quickly two fully constructed buildings for their future homes. When the first crisis came, in the form of a big bad wolf, what the two little pigs had built crumbled and did not survive. The third little pig invested his money and time and built a structure to last. When the same crisis confronted him, a well-built foundation helped avert disaster. He survived with the opportunity to thrive and prosper.

What the third little pig learned was that he should be prepared to meet unavoidable crisis situations.

The failure to utilize professional services at the outset of entering into a practice may result in a practice structure that may not survive crises with which it is confronted. Early employment of Practice Consultants' legal, accounting, banking and insurance services may, in fact, prevent crises down the road.

Many doctors, eager to find a suitable location for their practice, enter into a lease agreement thinking it is just a form document. They may be unaware that the "form" lease agreement is extremely favorable to the lessor.

Most lease agreements are negotiable at the outset but once executed, oppressive provisions may not come to light until a dispute arises later. You are urged to have an attorney review your lease and assist you in negotiating terms that would be favorable and fair to you and not just to the landlord.

Beginning a practice, you should use professional services as part of your cost of doing business from the outset, and these should be implicit in the above. Utilizing such services in the formative stages of business will usually be less expensive in the long run than using such services on a crisis management basis.

Undoubtedly, many young doctors ask the wrong question, mainly, "Can I afford a professional consultant?" The better question is, "Can I afford not to have professional services and lose the time and money investment which I have spent in obtaining my chiropractic education?"

TIPS ON BUILDING A SUCCESSFUL PRACTICE

1) Before opening your office, conduct a survey of a minimum of 400 to a maximum of 500 people on a one-to-one basis. Ask the following questions and write down all the answers:
   a. "I am considering opening a chiropractic office in this area. Do you think there is a need for such services?"
   b. "Have you or any of your relatives ever been to a chiropractor?" Write down the answer and if possible, find out who.
   c. "Where do you feel a chiropractor's office would be best suited to be located?"

   Get the name of the person you have interviewed, their address and phone number, and keep this information. Then, upon opening your office, write to them and thank them for encouraging you to open in their city. These people will become your referral team.

   It is much easier to use this approach than to open your office and anticipate an immediate influx of new patients.
2) Once you have chosen a location for your office, place a simple announcement in the paper stating that you will be opening on or about (date). State that advance appointments are now being taken and list your phone number. You can place a telephone recording service on the phone if you are out of the office and call the prospective patients back to set up an appointment.

50% OF YOUR SUCCESS IS DUE TO THESE FACTORS

Practice Consultants did extensive practice research

more than ten years ago and proved conclusively that 50% of a doctor's success was dependent upon an efficient, knowledgeable, and well-trained office manager (chiropractic assistant). In fact, Practice Consultants was the first management firm to insist that its clients bring their front desk office manager to every seminar that he/she might be trained in the skills of effectively answering the telephone. Our research revealed as many as 50% of prospective patients failed to make appointments because of poor telephone techniques in negotiating an appointment. The manager is also trained in collections, insurance skills, and creating a warm and friendly atmosphere in the office, and so forth. Always remember that patients go where they are invited and stay where they are recognized and appreciated.

Practice Consultants' research has revealed that it is to the ultimate benefit of the young practitioner to employ his/her spouse as a chiropractic assistant for the first years of the practice, provided the spouse has no hesitation in taking the position and has a pleasing, outgoing personality. If he/she feels unsuitable for this position, you are advised not to press the issue. Our experience has shown that if your spouse does assume this position initially, he/she will be able to learn the business side of the practice and in the future become, in fact, the office manager, able to train additional assistants. This relieves the doctor of the details which are usually not his/her talent and for which there is little time because of the patient load.

You should never, ever hire a person you cannot fire without abnormal stress. For example, friends and close relatives with few exceptions do not make good help and are very difficult to terminate if they become unsuited for the job. Simply by calling an employment service, you will be furnished with qualified applicants without charge to you.

The best employees are between the ages of 25 and 35. Make sure that all children, if any, are in school, thus eliminating the employee having to go home and attend a sick child and other complications.

A divorced person separated for six months or longer is ideal, providing the applicant is willing to attend seminars to increase office skills. Never employ a chiropractic assistant where there is not a firm understanding initially of this requirement. If the applicant is married, have this agreement, in person from his/her spouse, before employment is started.

A doctor who employs assistants who are not growing will not grow; they will retard the growth. Be aware of this always.

Be sure to read the employment form and to check very carefully the prospect's past employment personally with his/her supervisors. If he/she has had a history of changing jobs every six months to a year in the past, he/she will have the same eagerness to leave you in the same period of time - so beware. Call the past employers and state, "Mr. Jones, Mr./Ms. Smith gave you as a reference and anything that you reveal to me will be held in strictest confidence and will not be known to him/her as he/she has given many references regarding past employers."

If the situation were reversed, I would be happy to answer the following questions:

1) On a scale from 1 to 10, how would you rate his/her performance in your office?
2) Was he/she out because of sickness or other circumstances abnormally?
3) What was his/her attitude?
4) Did he/she work well with other employees?
5) Did you find him/her willing and eager to learn, or did he/she resist changes within your office?

6) Finally, what was his/her reason for leaving your employment and would you employ him/her again?" (Providing reasons given by employee were valid.)

So important is this field of placing the right person in the right position that Practice Consultants had one of our staff take extensive training in screening potential employees and selecting the right employee for the right position. This staff member counsels each doctor to make sure that he/she employs the most competent, capable person for the position to be filled.

During the interview with your prospect, determine if he/she has any reservations about collecting money. It is a proven fact that if the employee is not personally on sound financial ground, he/she will make a poor collector. This is because he/she will always relate to the circumstances of the patients who state that they are having a hard time making payments and so forth.

THE FINAL ADVICE

Your attitude - your commitment - is the key to ultimate success in any field you choose to pursue.

If your goal is to succeed in the chiropractic profession, be prepared to adopt an attitude of success by making a lasting commitment to yourself.

DR. HARRIS'
SEVEN STEPS TO CHIROPRACTIC SUCCESS

1) Immediately establish long-range and short-range goals in writing. Reach for the stars!
2) Hire staff carefully. Screen properly. Train thoroughly. Stress teamwork - your success depends upon a good staff.
3) Meet three new people a day. Tell them who you are and where you are. Hand out business cards. Meeting three new people a day keeps the blues away!
4) Continuously build your professional image in the community - market yourself.
5) Exercise daily to relieve stress - eat right.
6) Keep a positive mental attitude. Develop an attitude of gratitude!
7) Educate your community to believe in chiropractic.

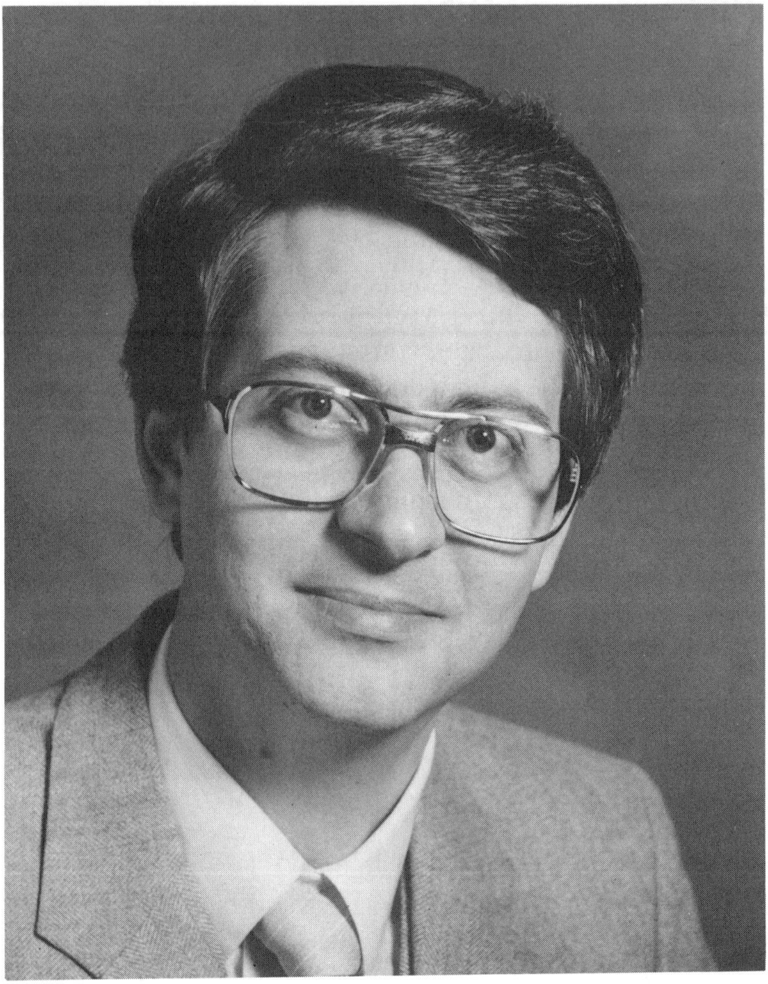

F. Michael Anderson, D.C.

F. MICHAEL ANDERSON, D.C.

ANDERSON MANAGEMENT SERVICES

Dr. F. Michael Anderson is co-founder of ANDERSON MANAGEMENT SERVICES along with Janice E. Anderson.

ANDERSON MANAGEMENT SERVICES was founded in 1982 as an alternative management company to serve the chiropractic profession without the standard management contract. AMS has two management programs: Practice Control for the chiropractor, and Staff Development Seminars for C.A. training. It is the purpose of AMS to provide in one-weekend workshops a total management package for total office growth, profitability and staff development. AMS provides a limited number of one-on-one ongoing monthly client positions for doctors needing the extra edge; this program is also low fee with no contract. AMS offers one of the foremost computer programs for the chiropractic office to aid in increased productivity. Within the first two years of ANDERSON MANAGEMENT SERVICES' existence, over 500 doctors and 2,000 chiropractic assistants were trained.

Seminar workshops are given often and regionally for the chiropractor's convenience. Information on upcoming seminars or client information may be received by writing:

ANDERSON MANAGEMENT SERVICES
23 Red Fox Run, Salisbury, North Carolina 28144
(704) 636-1272

NOTES / GOALS:

CHAPTER 2
The Steps to Practice Control

F. Michael Anderson, D.C.

Success in practice can be measured by many yardsticks. . . but whatever measurement is applied must be recognizable, both qualitatively and quantitatively. It must be an attainable, ethical and totally satisfying goal which you will recognize immediately when it arrives.

My personal picture of success can be described as: A practice which functions at the lowest possible level of stress for the doctors, the assistants and the patients.

A low-level stress office is one which functions smoothly without crisis interruptions, frantic questions to the doctor regarding routine matters and the orderly handling of financial data. The emphasis is on new patient acquisition, not routine chores which are assigned to responsible persons other than the doctor.

The doctor makes things happen. Ideally, he/she is in control of the total practice environment. And, a prime responsibility is the doctor's efforts to attract new patients, create a referral attitude within patients and oversee an orderly cash flow.

The doctor practices for the fun of practicing, not to meet the overhead. This is the concept which forms the heart of a program through which you can visualize and reach the goal of practice success. . .we call it simply, Practice Control. Here's how it can work for you.

PRACTICE CONTROL

Practice Control means just that. . .you control your office with all its major and minor functions.

Stress is a key factor in a doctor's emotional and physical ability to develop and maintain a successful practice. If you can develop and maintain control of your practice, then the stress level imposed upon everyone decreases. With stress contained within a comfort zone, the practice is more likely to nurture and grow to its fullest potential . . .to the ultimate goals you have projected.

Essentially, there are four primary phases of concern which will help you to understand more fully the implication of being in total charge of all the inner workings of your office. These four phases are: 1) Patient Control, 2) Staff Development, 3) Staff Management and 4) Practice Control.

STEPS TO GAINING CONTROL

To be in command, the doctor must relay as much information to the patient as possible during the first few minutes to the first few days. This information must cover financial policies, report of findings and patient education.

We're often asked during our seminar meetings what is the biggest obstacle doctors experience with implementing Practice Control ideas. The straightforward answer is: "Reaching the realization that true growth and success come from having an office procedure that plugs all the leaks in the practice. It is procedure which keeps patients happy and educated, which, in turn, means follow through with care. This results in frequent referrals."

Many doctors strive for a "quick fix" which will reflect quick growth, right now. Of course, there are some isolated examples of this, but generally the "quick fix" has many drawbacks. If the practice does not have the holes plugged, then new growth is lost. The practice continues its roller coaster syndrome causing the doctor frustration.

These pitfalls can be eliminated in your practice by following the outlined suggestions presented both in this chapter and throughout *Seven Steps to Chiropractic Success.* You'll awaken to face an office day without stress, distress or avoidable aggravation . . . and that's always a wonderful feeling! Also, you'll experience more profitable stability and honest growth.

FINANCIAL POLICIES

Undoubtedly one of the major factors that can cause hard feelings between the patient and the doctor is the lack of a written financial policy. A written financial policy is a simple straightforward list of payment options that the patient has for paying for the services rendered in your office. It is ideal that this form be handed to the patient in the reception room after greeting. For example, "Mrs. Jones, Dr. Anderson would like you to fill out our patient introductory form totally, and then read over our office financial policy. Bring the introductory form to the front desk when you are finished with it; you may keep the financial policy."

It is not necessary for the patient to sign or return this form unless you have a collection problem in your area. Having the patient read this prior to the consultation removes any preconceived ideas they may have concerning payment. If there are any problems, then they can be covered prior to any services being rendered. This up-front presentation of your payment regulations helps to free you to concentrate on the patient's health.

Remember, however, a written financial policy is just that, rules for the doctor to be paid. You must dispel the impression that "Well, the patient's health is number one to me, the money is secondary." This may be true, but when the patient's account gets out of hand, you become annoyed and aggravated and your bills begin to slide. You share the responsibility to see whatever agreements are entered into are duly performed. If they're not, someone must accept blame for lack of responsibility. This could be a mighty significant leak in any office.

Be realistic! How long can you continue to see patients if you have no income?

For example, one of my clients before attending our workshop had Accounts Receivable of over $80,000 in an office collecting $10,000-$15,000 monthly. We recommend your A/R not exceed two times monthly gross services. Upon evaluating this client's office, we found no written policy regarding financial obligations. The major weakness was the doctor failed to pre-advise the patient of how the patient could pay and that payment was expected. While hope does spring eternal, it's a poor way to effect collection of money you need to build your future and stay free of stress because your obligations are current.

Fortunately, his problems were correctable. He applied our formulae of Practice Control and dropped his A/R to

$30,000 within sixty days. Within six months he found his A/R staying within a comfortable 1½ times his monthly service gross. How? Using written financial policies.

Another variation of this problem area is the "Chiropractic Missionary" complex. This is similar to the above example but has this variation. The patient tells a hard-luck story and the doctor offers to treat the patient with payment "when you can." Once the patient is dismissed, the doctor becomes aggravated that the patient is not paying the bill. In other words, he/she has forgotten the original agreement. Our advice to avoid this: If you adopt the "Missionary" role, continue it throughout the treatment period and don't begrudge your losses. To make demands or requests for payment places stress upon patient, yourself and your staff. It's difficult to "close-end" an already "open-ended" contract without some disagreement. This procedure also creates staff confusion and resentment toward you, their leader.

Your first rule to follow should be: Have a definite written financial policy - and follow it without exceptions. It should be simple and explicit.

To write a workable policy, enumerate all the methods available and acceptable to you for payment:

1) CASH
2) INSURANCE: If you accept this form of payment, list your rules for this procedure and what is expected from the patient, your billing Chiropractic Assistant (CA), etc. Always have the patient supply the appropriate claim form or sign a standard AMA-approved claim form prior to accepting assignment. Advise the patient that they are responsible for any unpaid portions not paid by their insurance company.
3) CHARGING SERVICES: The only credit provisions, or charging, we recommend is the use of charge cards

. . .which gets you paid that day.

4) WORKER'S COMPENSATION: This may vary from state to state. Nevertheless, let the patient know what the financial facts are before starting treatment.

5) PERSONAL INJURY: This also varies in different states, especially those with "No Fault" limitations. Make certain you have all required liens, both attorney and insurance, before starting your program. Never proceed with treatment without a clear-cut written agreement from the patient to pay you, and any attorneys, if applicable. When in doubt, have the patient pay cash until a legitimate verifiable means of getting paid is in your hands.

   Always investigate the patient's policy for MED-Pay and contact the insurance carrier for a claim number. A simple printed policy which is given to the patient and signed by them eliminates any possibility for misunderstanding of your personal injury policy.

Again, the ideal time to present your written policy is during the patient's first visit when they receive your patient introduction form. You'll find most of your financial problems will vanish if this is accomplished at this time. A reminder: Once you have established a written financial policy, you must use this consistently with each patient.

REPORT OF FINDINGS

This is one of the most important phases of the doctor/ patient relationship. It establishes several landmarks which will be used throughout the patient's association with your office.

First, your report to the patient outlines their problems and what program will be utilized to correct these problems. You may summarize their condition in both oral and written form, preferably on their second visit.

The points you should cover are: X-ray and physical examination findings, and your overall plan for solution of their problems.

The written report should cover what chiropractic is, additional examination findings, rehabilitation exercises, types of care you offer, what treatment is recommended and all financial information the patient can utilize to cover their projected treatment program. It is not necessary or recommended to have the patient sign this written report.

No guarantee should be offered or implied. A written report, according to most doctors, seems to carry more weight and encourages better follow-through by the patient than only an oral report. It also prompts payment at scheduled times.

What are the relative merits of a planned treatment program vs. an unplanned method of care?

The doctor who does not offer planned care is, basically, treating symptoms. These patients can be expected to be discharged after 1-10 visits. If the patient has any degree of spinal degeneration, this rationale will be inadequate for total health welfare. Also, this doctor must see a high volume of new patients just to survive.

On the other hand, patients who clearly understand the concept of spinal degeneration and subluxation complex are those most likely to refer others to their caring doctor and to follow through with enthusiasm their assigned schedule of treatment. This produces a more stable and stronger practice, and accounts for ultimate success.

Another vital point is patient education . . . it goes hand-in-hand with a smoothly running office.

Dr. Brown presents a classic example. When first we met at our seminar, Dr. Brown had an 18-visit patient retention. His attitude was, "I felt as though I had to beg patients to come in, and when they did, they just didn't – or wouldn't – follow through with weekly suggested visits based on how they were feeling. The moment they felt a little better, they were gone."

We remedied Dr. Brown's weaknesses by advising written reports, no exceptions, no excuses. While it seemed harsh at first, it wasn't long before the magic began... within eight weeks his average visit retention jumped to 29 visits and is still climbing. Dr. Brown says, "The patients now do exactly what I tell them...and referrals are up...what a happy relief!"

PATIENT EDUCATION

As mentioned previously, this is an especially sensitive and important area of practice responsibility.

Recognize the two principal types of care you can provide patients: 1) Relief care and 2) Corrective/stabilization care.

Relief care is designed to relieve the patient's immediate pain. This is fairly close to "aspirin therapy." It makes a person immediately happy, but it travels only a short distance toward a condition of total health. Also, it places little importance on the etiologic factors which may have contributed to the "sudden" strain/sprain injury the patient experienced. It is usually the tire with uneven tire wear that blows out, not the new, well-balanced one.

Corrective/stabilization care should be thoroughly explained through the variety of educational processes at your disposal. From this, the patient understands – frequently demands – that this is the avenue of care they want to follow. "I don't ever want this to happen again," is a common expression by the emergency patient who realizes what has happened to them might have been prevented had certain measures been taken in advance of their painful experience. How right they are.

Teaching the complexities of subluxation is covered extensively in each of our seminars. Our reasoning is even though you may understand all the factors, we each must be reminded that the patient is not of a professional background. . . it's news to them and they are the ones who need this basic understanding to structure their life free of illness and backache.

I found the Renaissance International Symposium an inspirational source to bring all the facets of subluxation complex into focus. We recommend our clients seek this "born again" motivational force to get their thinking back on track. Understanding subluxation and spinal degeneration is the first major key for both the doctor and patient to give and follow through with care.

Once you have applied either a video, written or spinal care lecture to bring patients up to a greater level of chiropractic understanding, the quicker you will embrace all the facets of successful chiropractic in your office.

DEVELOPING THE IDEAL STAFF

Remember the old saying, "Without a nail the shoe was lost, and without a shoe the horse was lost"? Don't lose the power of your office because your staff lacks the horsepower to provide a smoothly functioning office. Also, remember, you are the leader. . . those who surround you must follow your lead, not the other way around.

To lead your staff, you must understand what you want them to accomplish. You must assign responsibility, that's your task.

The staff should function like clockwork: smart, organized, loyal and dedicated to your success.

The job starts at the hiring level. . .you must hire the right person for the particular job. . . it may be a challenge, but there is a way to accomplish this without undue stress.

Write a job description before interviewing applicants so that both the doctor and the applicant know what the job entails. You must have a clear picture of what is needed before you can recognize the right person when they appear. The following are our requirements for a front office assistant: 1) Typing skills: 40 WPM, 2) 10-key adding machine touch, 3) Hours, 4) Benefits, 5) Vacations, 6) Test all applicants you would consider hiring to determine their exact proficiency. Find out their pluses or minuses before they start working for you.

If the applicant has no problems with the above (be honest about your office hours), we use an oral interview to determine degree of motivation, and personality compatibility before making a final decision.

Training the new-hire is the next important step toward putting an office staff into place. We find the buddy-system of having a CA train the new staff member works well. However, skip this if the departing CA is a less than happy individual. Make certain there is adequate time provided to read through your training manual and all questions about your procedures are fully explained in the beginning, otherwise, the new employee may feel the training manual accounts for little and will tend to ignore it in the future.

The new CA's first day should be split between observing and doing. During morning hours he/she can follow the experienced CA, then reverse the procedure during the afternoon. Repeat this for the next 2-3 days until he/she demonstrates familiarity with all required duties. In our experience, within two weeks the new CA will have the "right stuff." If this guideline is not working, the doctor would be well advised to reexamine the new CA's qualifications.

USE A PROCEDURAL MANUAL

Following the instructions contained in a procedural manual allows every staff member to have a clear understanding of what's expected and avoids repeated discussion regarding areas of discontent.

This booklet should be written with staff input so it is concise and complete. Update it frequently. It should describe in detail how each duty is to be performed, by whom, and when. It is the beginning point for developing proper staff management. Also, it has the positive feature of measuring performance, which is valuable for receiving rewards for a job well done. If you have written in black and white what is expected, you are on your way to proper staff management. The procedural manual is ideal for cross-training staff in the event of vacations or other times when the office is understaffed.

STAFF MANAGEMENT

The single most important ingredient in putting together a smoothly functioning office staff is the consistent display of strong leadership qualities by the doctor.

We polled several offices to determine the needs of CAs and found it wasn't salary that was number one; it was leadership they wanted. The people who work with you want a boss who recognizes when a job is well done and who gives credit for a record of excellent work performance.

In the final analysis, this translates into good communication between the doctor and staff. There is very little discussion when responsibilities are clearly assigned and frequent meetings allow airing of any unresolved problem areas. Also, this allows the doctor the opportunity to show appreciation for reaching practice goals.

STAFF POLICIES

The first step toward reaching desirable staff management and an efficiently functioning office is creating an office policy manual.

This manual should include the following:

1) Introduction to Chiropractic
2) General CA Attitude
3) Office Appearance and Uniforms
4) Salary Reviews and Promotions
5) Employee Benefits and Vacations
6) Office Policies and Regulations

Each employee should familiarize themselves with this manual, and the doctor should not deviate or make exceptions in following the written rules, which have been accepted by staff members in writing.

PRODUCTION LOGS

There are several ways to measure practice growth and performance. One of the most effective means is through various written schedules - production logs - which show data concerning areas of patient acquisition, cash flow and overhead, plus several other critical factors which lead to a stress-free practice.

The point to keep in mind is, your time should be reserved for healing people, not engaging in routine chores. When the necessary data is compiled daily through the appropriate logs, you spend only a minimum time to oversee each office function.

Therefore, entering information daily into the logs should be assigned to the CA responsible for that particular area. Verbal communication regarding stats should be avoided, as this information relies upon memorization, a time-consuming and haphazard method of data keeping.

Written reports keep you in control, a key element in office leadership.

A classic example which highlights the lesson of maintaining adequate written logs is the case of Dr. Jones. He was totally baffled as to why he was constantly busy, but there was never enough money. Added to this, he needed more new patients even though his office was constantly full and busy. When we inquired as to certain records and office statistics, he replied, "Oh, I don't worry about that . . . the staff takes care of all the details. I just want to adjust patients, the CAs can take care of the front office." They were taking care of it all right, but not in any manner which benefited Dr. Jones!

We found - after an extensive period of reconstruction of past financial records - his A/R sky high, six months his production. Patient retention was extremely low, even though his reports were excellent. Missed appointments, we found, were never contacted; this was the patient's responsibility?? The CA responsible for collections would ask the patients if they wanted to pay today. And, of course, nobody did!

Today Dr. Jones never lets a day go by without checking the front desk for a complete review of all the daily logs. Needless to say, he's in control now and the practice reflects it with an almost current cash flow and an organized team of assistants.

Many doctors are lost when it comes time to evaluate a staff person's performance. We are often asked, "How do I base whether I give someone a raise or not?" There are many criteria, but only two will be covered at this time. First, is attitude. Unfortunately, you cannot judge this on paper, but you can by observing the staff person. Therefore, you do not need a log for staff attitude. However, if you have logs that each staff person maintains according to the duties he/she performs, then you have at your disposal a means to grade whether a raise is appropriate at a particular time. If the logs are filled out properly and totally for each employee, then you know that he/she is doing the work. Then, it is a matter of simply basing a raise on performance and attitude. Maintaining staff production logs is one way you become a good staff manager. The next area will contribute to better doctor/staff communication.

THE POWER OF COMMUNICATION

Staff meetings should be a two-way street . . . the meeting of minds of doctor and staff. A well-planned staff meeting can improve overall cooperation, increase office loyalty and produce practice growth. They don't have to end on a sour note . . . if the doctor keeps an open mind and provides leadership with fair decisions and appreciation of consistent performance.

A staff meeting should never become a gripe session . . . it should provide solutions which eliminate discontent and encourages total motivation to attain office and practice goals. It helps to keep the discussion centered on improved patient relations and better traffic control, rather than personal disputes or gripes. Review patient progress or lack of progress and ask for suggestions to improve whatever is determined a weakness in procedure or attitude.

A staff meeting should strive to fire up enthusiasm by the entire staff. Engage an emotional, rather than logical, overtone to help each staff member visualize the Big Picture. These are the steps to create harmony and growth.

A meeting should be held at least weekly, even though it might be brief and direct. Establish the habit within the office of knowing there is a time and place for everything. . . including discussion. It is best not to allow interruptions during the staff meeting period. Don't engage a staff person in conversation which can be better handled privately.

REACHING YOUR GOALS

Your ultimate aim in practice is to reach your goals. We believe sincerely every doctor can attain any goal through a program of Practice Control. . . the creation of an efficient office environment.

Keeping your mind open to new ideas is a mental procedure and attitude that the successful doctor always has as part of his/her personality. Open-mindedness means getting rid of practice prejudices, harmful old habits, a willingness to consider or experience alternate growth subjects as opposed to your present mind-set, and attachment to procedures which seem set in concrete. There's a world of variety to look at: New adjusting techniques, X-ray and imaging techniques, treatment and diagnostic approaches, practice building methods, and staff management innovations. The successful doctors have one characteristic in common: They attend many, many educational seminars or postgraduate courses in the health and business aspect of the office.

Another necessary ingredient to reaching your established goal is staff watchfulness . . . keeping one eye on the store at all times. Inattention breeds discontent, fraud and a totally false picture of what's going on in your practice . . . it's the hallmark of a poor manager, and a red flag calling attention to the lack of practice control.

As doctors, we like the feeling of personal independence . . . of being "our own man." Why, then, does an intelligent, skillful, and thoughtful individual allow a less trained, less dedicated person take over the reins of an operation he/she has financed, nurtured and worked hard and long to build? And, allow this to happen believing he/she won't have to pay the consequences sooner or later for his/her indifference to vital conditions of the practice?

The surest way to reach your goals is through consistency and determination to adhere to basic rules of business conduct . . . your rules, to be sure, but rules to be followed, without exception.

LET PEOPLE KNOW WHO YOU ARE

We're not too concerned with the differences between Public Relations and Advertising . . . the principle is: Let People Know Who You Are. We buy from friends, so become the best friend in your community.

How many strangers have you talked to today? last week? last month? Sit in your local shopping mall and see how many people you know by name who walk by . . . these are all potential friends, if you make the effort to meet them. Count the many ways available to let them know who you are, and where you are when they need you.

Good public relations needn't cost an arm or leg. You can start your program in your office by being happy and enthusiastic. . . this is the type of friend each of us wants to know better, they are a joy to associate with. As Dr. Jim Parker says, "ACT AS IF. . ." and let this image flow from your office into the community.

Another means of attracting attention to your office is through education, using in-house video, newsletters or spinal care classes. Let people know what you do and how you do it so well.

The patient newsletter has a very significant purpose. Believe it or not, patients do not think of you between visits. At least, not continually. You may be a great doctor and have a wonderful, charming personality, but patients have lives to lead, too. It is for this reason that you must continually have a system to remind patients that you exist and that chiropractic is a necessary part of their lives and the lives of others whom they come in contact with daily.

It is our recommendation to send out a patient newsletter every three weeks. I would make sure that my patients knew who I was, and what benefit chiropractic had for them and anyone they know with a spine. Many doctors work their practice like they would a slot machine in Las Vegas. They put a quarter in a slot machine and pray for the $25,000 jackpot. It rarely happens. Many doctors are burned out, selling shoes or insurance, or have a mediocre practice from lack of practice effort in the public relations field. Think about this – if McDonald's and Coca Cola think it is important to advertise or inform the public of what they have available, and everyone knows their names, then why is it some chiropractors think that just being open will bring practice success? Why wait for years for your name to be known or connected with chiropractic, and even then to only a small percentage of your community? You must decide that whether you decide on low-key public relations, spinal care classes, community newsletters, or full coverage public relations that your community will know your name and what you have to offer.

I believe you can agree that two of the basic requirements for success are:

1) Keep an open mind
2) Be consistent

OFFICE CAPACITY

This is a term frequently misunderstood by many doctors. Capacity has held back more doctors from the next stage of growth than any other single practice stepping stone.

Capacity means using the space you have to its maximum potential. . . the physical layout of your office and the routine traffic flow through your office.

Many doctors feel that in order to grow, a monument to chiropractic is required. The evidence doesn't support this, in fact, I know several doctors seeing a minimum of 1,200 visits per month – with incomes ranging from $60-$200,000 monthly – who have no more than 800-1,400 square feet of office space. It's not uncommon for the busiest doctors to utilize the smallest of offices.

There are certain keys to phenomenal growth and income in relationship to capacity. The first is utilizing one or two adjustment rooms for treatment. The doctor who goes from treatment room to treatment room is not only stressing himself, but self-limiting his/her practice. Why? The simple logistics of walking from room to room, which accounts for 30 seconds. Multiplying all this walking time, the doctor finds 30 minutes of every day is lost from adjusting just in traveling time from room to room. The office with two adjustment rooms, one being only for acute patients, and two examination rooms is primed for growth. Or, the super-functional arrangement of examination room serving as an acute-consult-report and first adjustment room.

Therapy is most efficiently used in a community therapy room. This method utilizes the least amount of staff, thus reducing your overhead.

The most efficiently run offices locate the adjustment room near the front desk and reception room area.

FINANCIAL INDEPENDENCE

The doctor who goes to the office each morning with the contented feeling this is what they want to do - not because they have to - is the person most likely to reach the goal of financial independence.

Overwhelming debt puts the doctor in the position of going to the office just to make ends meet, and this attitude reflects onto patients. . .you have a job not a career.

There are two successful methods to reach financial goals. First, you must begin to accumulate money. Second, follow a capable financial management program (we highly recommend the Whitehall Seminars).

Don't be discouraged, this is the key to opening windows to turn your present practice and professional career into a flourishing and stress-free lifestyle. It is possible to practice ethically, legally, enthusiastically with moderate volume and accumulate $500,000 in cash and retire within five to ten years.

You begin this journey by taking the first steps . . . the steps you have in *Seven Steps to Chiropractic Success* . . . the secret is, reach out for what is yours!

List your goals and the action steps which take you to your destination. Now, go for it.

DR. ANDERSON'S
SEVEN STEPS TO CHIROPRACTIC SUCCESS:

1) Develop a written policy for the entire office that spells out the "hows," "whys" and "what ifs" for your practice.
2) Educate every patient.
3) Develop and manage your staff to their fullest potential.
4) Be consistent in all practice areas.
5) Be THE chiropractor in your area.
6) Prepare for your financial independence today.
7) Believe you can - and you will.

NOTES / GOALS:

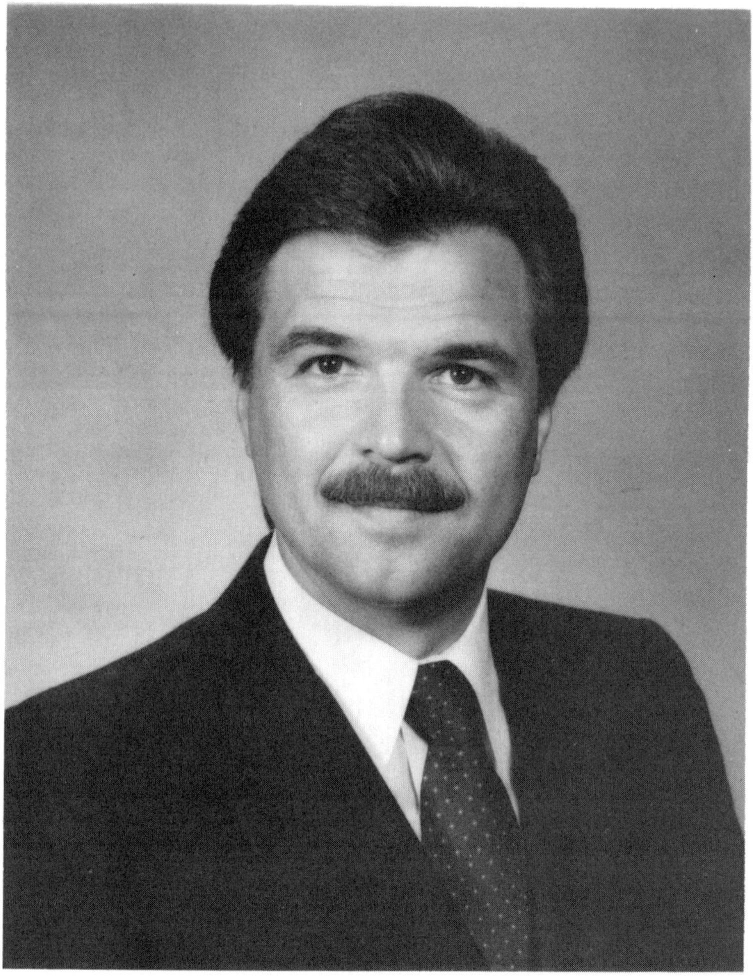

Micheil Hanczaryk, D.C.

MICHEIL HANCZARYK, D.C.

It cannot be overemphasized that management consultants and the skills they teach are in no way a substitution for the final product.

In chiropractic, it is the doctor's ability to examine, diagnose, treat and eliminate the subluxation from the spine. We in no way condone unethical practices. All management skills are taught to support the doctor's diagnosis and treatment plan.

Management skills only complement what the patient needs - not what the doctor needs.

The management ideas presented in this chapter are in no way to be misinterpreted as a substitution for good, honest chiropractic treatment when it comes to the needs of the patient. We always consider what the patient needs - not what the doctor thinks he needs.

The bottom line is results, and in the patient's case, that's health free of subluxation. This is, of course, based on thorough consultation, examination, X-ray, and treatment as taught in our chiropractic colleges.

MICHEIL HANCZARYK, D.C.
5098 W. Bristol, Flint, Michigan 48507
(313) 733-1261

NOTES / GOALS:

CHAPTER 3
Getting to the Top – and Staying There

Micheil Hanczaryk, D.C.

What's wrong with being the best you can be?

If your answer is "Nothing," this chapter can lead you up the steps to greater professional attainment; but, it isn't a substitute for honest, ethical and skillful practice technique.

You've got to evaluate, diagnose and treat the patient with a high degree of satisfactory results. You learned this in chiropractic college and through technique seminars. However, total success requires more than just good chiropractic adjustments.

It requires the identical skills in business management to reach to top and stay there. And, this is how *Seven Steps to Chiropractic Success* can help you put both segments of your career into focus and lead you to the top.

Why am I so confident you have the ability to learn and apply good management techniques and procedures? Because, I, too, have traveled the same road, experienced similar frustrations and put my nose to the same grindstone you have.

If my story can shed some light on where I get my drive to build a high-level practice during extremely adverse economic periods of the late 70's and 80's – in Flint, Michigan, no less – then I know you're getting an honest value from this book.

Let's start at the beginning . . .

I was born of Ukrainian immigrants who possess a deeply embedded faith in God and the Work Ethic. I was taught I could be anything I wanted, if I wanted it badly enough . . . and was willing to work hard enough to get it.

I was impressed with the parable: Give a man a fish and he will eat for a day. Teach a man to fish, and he will eat for a lifetime.

I can state proudly that my parents taught me to fish . . . thanks, Mom and Dad. They also taught me to have dreams and visions, as in Neil Diamond's song, "America":

"We've been traveling far without a home,
but not without a star.
Free. Only want to be free –
we huddle close, hang onto a dream.
On the boats and on the planes they come into America.
Never looking back again, they're coming to America.
Home. Doesn't it seem so far away?
We're traveling light today in the eye of a storm . . .
home to a new and shining place.
Make our bed and say our grace.
Freedom's light burning warm.
They're coming to America,
gotta dream to take 'em there."

Yes, we came over on the boat some years ago to make a fresh start in America. Green as grass, but burning with desire.

Recently, while vacationing with my wife and children, we flew into Los Angeles, rented a car and headed for San Diego. Although hungry and tired, I came alive when I saw a sign, "Long Beach - Queen Mary." As if a magnet pulled me, I swung off the freeway and parked the car where I could see her, the Queen. What a magnificent sight for a former passenger, a perfect reunion after 31 years.

As I walked her decks, my mind went back to our passage... I only then fully realized the courage my parents must have had to sell all their possessions and sail to a new land. What apprehension they must have experienced landing in New York with not much more than hope and a four-year-old. But, in contrast to their experiences in WW II Nazi war camps, America did look good, and proved later to be a wonderful blessing.

So, you see I was born with great hopes and expectations... and a willingness to work, learn and put my shoulder to the wheel to become the best I could. Choosing chiropractic as a vehicle to get there was also just good luck... to choose such a wonderfully satisfying profession was a never-ending blessing.

One other factor I learned about success... just being a good doctor isn't a complete formula, it takes being a good manager, too, to complete the equation... and this is where this book can help you. Just as you strive to excel with treatment procedures, you've got to join the other half - office procedures - to make a wholly successful career.

MANAGEMENT OVERVIEW

At the top of the best seller lists today are books which deal with people - how to move ahead and maintain your sanity, your family, and your innerself. In other words, progress and yet smell the roses along the way. Other writings go along the vein of management, books such as "What They Don't Teach at Harvard Business School," "In Search of Excellence," and "The One Minute Manager" which has developed into "The One Minute Mother and the One Minute Father."

Even though this country has excelled and been the world leader in almost all endeavors, it took a small country the size of Japan to wake us up from the sleep of medicority. What I speak of is not what happened to just the automobile industry in the late 1970's and early 1980's, but to all businesses and industry. We found Japan beating us at our own game. There are many opinions and countless books written as to why. The one I want to concentrate on primarily is management.

There seems to be a certain mystique surrounding that class of individuals known as "management." Everyone, of course, is a manager to some extent for we are all in charge of our lives and it takes a certain something to be willing to take charge of a group of employees.

Working with people to make an organization reach an objective and have them get some satisfaction from it is exciting and fulfilling.

People who win great battles or make a lot of money have a vision of what's required for victory and they find a realistic way of making that vision come true. The people you have around you can - and will - add to your success or failure.

If you study the lives of great leaders throughout history and the present, you'll discover these individuals didn't accomplish things on a solo basis. These individuals learned early the art of surrounding themselves with experts in their field. In other words - don't try being an expert in everything. Don't be your own accountant, attorney, investment advisor or management consultant. Be a true entrepreneur - use the experience of others in harmony with your own specialty if you expect to set the pace in your profession.

You may be of the opinion that all you want to do is be a professional, and practice your particular discipline of health care. Such statements as "All I want to do is be a chiropractor," "If only all the other hassels would go away I would be just fine," are heard over and over when consulting with clients. Ben Franklin once said, "Run thy business or thy business will run you." The reality of the situation is this: The problems will never go away, you are the only one that can hold the reins of control and growth of your practice. Your practice, of course, is to get people well through chiropractic, but in the same breath, you run a business - a people and health business. The bottom line is you must have a profit or you no longer exist. You can be the greatest chiropractor in the world, but if you can't keep your doors open it's all useless.

General George S. Patton, Jr. once said, "Issuing an order is worth 10%. The remaining 90% consists in assuring proper and vigorous execution of the order."

I like to feel my experiences gained in building a seven-figure chiropractic practice qualifies me to be a "management consultant." Also, I like to feel my desire to help others reach their full potential through moral and ethical procedures is a satisfying personal goal.

Having clients at various levels of success in practice, brings the opportunity to take a mediocre practice and turn it into a growing and thriving practice . . . and also taking a high-level practice and smoothing out the problems associated with running a high-level practice - things such as staff training, staying on purpose, time and money management, preventing burnout and becoming financially independent. And, of course, the major of majors is: "How do you continue to enjoy clinical growth and maintain a dynamic family relationship?" What good is all the success in your career if you lose your family along the way?

And lastly, I have seen many colleagues reach a high degree of success one day, month or year, and in the next moment fall to the bottom. As many of you will or have discovered, it's a challenge to get to the top, but it's very difficult to maintain that high caliber of practice growth. And so the roller coaster practice starts to take shape as the practice extracts an unbearable toll. Many a corporate president or C.E.O. has said getting to the top is relatively easy compared to staying there.

Many chiropractors seem to think that with a higher degree of success the problems will go away. Not so!! They only get more complicated and more numerous. In most instances, I find the chiropractor has not grown personally as fast as the practice. The primary area of deficiency is in the doctor's management skills. So, the practice slips.

Initially, we train a client and his/her staff in all facets of office procedures, then we add to this with management skills to keep the practice and doctor green and growing.

Chiropractic is not that different from any other major corporation. Our needs and wants are very similar. What works at G.M., I.B.M., and Chrysler applies in our own mini-corporation. Procedures help get you there and sustain a certain level of success, but it's your management skills that will get you into the major leagues. No longer do you – the owner/operator – have to take all the blame and do all the directing. The staff can learn what we call participant management versus passive management. The entire staff is actively involved, accountable, and responsible for the growth of the practice.

Good management helps you provide the best services to the most number of patients in the most efficient and cost-effective manner.

Those who profess to practice without growing or caring are only actors on an empty stage - unseen, unlistened to, unfeeling, and unrewarded by either applause or self-respect.

Management consists of promoting people and products. When health professionals initially start their practices they focus on being a chiropractor, optometrist, dentist, etc. But as the practice grows they find that they must also - and I emphasize also, not in lieu of - now become managers. Practices that initially grow and then taper off suffer from a lack of management skills. The professional feels if he/she becomes involved in management that he/she suddenly becomes less of a health care provider.

The facts of life are that you have been managed by someone all of your life - your parents, teachers, or bosses. All careers eventually lead to management and management means people.

Skill, hard work and dedication early in a career gets you just so far. It is difficult to "get to the top" on the basis of technical competence alone. Over-reliance on technical skills and neglect of the people skills leads to a leveling-off effect. To continue to advance, the people skills of the manager are needed to get the product out to the masses. There are no tricks to being a manager - just an awareness to respond to the human needs of your staff. Outstanding managers, parents and teachers share several characteristics which gain the acceptance and respect of those they supervise. They are the tools of management which lead the way, but not necessarily the easy way.

Often I have been accused of being very driven and to

a degree I must admit that is the case – especially when it comes to management and people. Basically, you cannot change an individual. You can't put something in people they do not already possess.

When I see an individual with potential I become very driven not so much to make the person a success, because only they can do that. But the drive comes in showing a person their potential and developing a belief in themselves. I figure if I can do that, then I have accomplished my objective and that individual will find his/her level of success. You can't push anyone – you can only pull them.

General Eisenhower once demonstrated to a group of army brass this principle: by placing a string on his desk he grasped one end of the string and attempted to push it. All it did was buckle up and gain no ground. Then, taking the same string he pulled it and, of course, it followed right along. So it is with people and management skills.

ADVICE TO FOLLOW

The following are points to remember when you work with people:

1) All people are motivated.
2) People do things for *their* reasons not for *yours*.
3) You cannot motivate people.
4) You can create factors which will be motivational in the environment.
5) People won't change for you but they may change with you.
6) If I know you, I may influence you.

Management means people!

SPINAL HEALTH CARE CLASS

"Trust in the future - it shall not betray you. These are good times if we but know what to do with them."

— Emerson

This quote by Emerson was my saving grace in the early stages of my practice and still offers a guiding light.

Being reared in Flint, Michigan, the birthplace of the automotive industry, as a young child I saw the tremendous rise and growth of General Motors and with it the hopes and futures of countless families which were dependent on the automobile. Sixty miles to the south is Detroit which was dependent on Ford, Chrysler and G.M. as well.

Michigan was dependent on the auto industry and enjoyed unprecedented prosperity. But in the late 1970's, along with Michigan, the rest of the nation soon realized the importance of the automotive industry in America. It is estimated that one in four jobs in the U.S. is in some way tied to the automobile. Suddenly one in four jobs was being lost due to the recession. Some say that in Michigan it was more like a depression. Thousands were left without jobs and futures. Faced with uncertainty, thousands fled the Midwest. On the Michigan-Indiana border someone erected a billboard which read, "Last one out turn out the lights." Such was the environment in Michigan.

Flint, which enjoyed the third highest per capita income of all the cities in the U.S., now became the number one unemployment capital of the entire nation. Flint has been given the distinction of being the host city of the recession of the 70's and 80's. This was the reality of the situation where I lived and set up practice in 1976.

P.M.A., or Positive Mental Attitude, can overcome many things, but all the P.M.A. in the world would not eliminate the reality of the hour. I'm sure the Chrysler corporation had many positive thinkers, but in 1979 they recorded an all-time corporate record loss and bankruptcy was inevitable. Something had to be done. Lee Iacocca totally restructured and met the enemy head-on. He formed a plan and worked the plan.

All the P.M.A. in the world will not keep you from getting wet when it rains outside if you go out unprepared. To prevent yourself from getting wet, use an umbrella – "an umbrella of protection." So, too, with the reality of the economy in Flint.

Many chiropractors and professionals chose not to participate in the recession but became victims due to the lack of preparation. They forgot their umbrellas.

My umbrella of protection in my practice became the spinal health care class. As the recession and unemployment grew out of control in Flint, our practice continued to enjoy unprecedented growth. On July 5, 1979, we broke ground for our 6,200-square-foot clinic and on December 6, 1979, we moved out of our 850-square-foot clinic into the new one. During the building phase the interest on the construction money was at 23.5%.

At this moment you are probably wondering what is the point of this? How can a spinal health care class offer an umbrella of protection for my practice? That's easy. Over 55% of all my new patients were directly derived from spinal health care class. And since most chiropractors are always starving for new patients, this would fulfill this need.

I would like to emphasize that new patients are not the key to a successful practice, but a lack of new patients offers no stability either. It's learning to manage what you now have.

Besides obtaining new patients, what is the purpose of

having spinal health care class? First and foremost, it is the doctor's obligation to diagnose or analyze, treat or adjust, and, lastly, to educate his patients. Next is what it does for the chiropractor himself. . . reaffirming his/her purpose. Also:

- Educated and informed patients follow through better
- Minimizes the negative influence of others
- Educates them in the do's and don'ts of proper spinal care
- Cost effective when compared to paying for advertising for new patients
- Time effective when educating several new patients at once
- Group support
- Understanding of what chiropractic is.

Many chiropractors have failing practices and yet do not spend the time to educate their patients. They say, "I know that already," but to know and not to do is not to know. They are afraid of doing a bad job. However, the worst lecture in the world is better than none at all. That reminds me of a couple of kids sitting on a curb and the one says to the other, "We didn't lose the game, we just didn't show up." Are you showing up when it comes to educating your patients?

There are four key factors to making spinal health care class a success.

1) The Commitment

After the report of findings is complete and the schedule of care is explained, the commitment to attend the class is obtained with the following dialogue.

"Mr. Subluxation, in order for us to accept your case, you must agree to come to the spinal care class. It's free, lasts for one hour and you only need to attend once. In the class we discuss things that will help you get better quicker – such as exercise, do's and don'ts of proper spinal care. . ." Ask them, "Do I have your commitment?"

Wait for a favorable response. Ninety percent of them will give you a positive response. Give them a ticket for the class with the date and time of the class.

2) The Class Itself

This is to last no longer than one hour, and consists of:

- Purpose and goal of the class
- Do's and don'ts while under care
- Exercise and its role in keeping you well
- Spinal anatomy
  Correlate the skeletal, neurological and organic relationship. Include a discussion of the life force (just like electricity).
- Medical tests to confirm this: E.M.G.; E.C.G.; E.E.G.
- Discussion of relief vs. care (include drugs and their effects).
- X-rays. Show before and after X-rays and scoliosis cases.

3) The Close of the Class

This is the most important part of the class and consists of three parts.

A. The personal story of either yourself, a family member, or a patient who was helped through chiropractic. The key is to make it or say it with emotional appeal. Remember well: people make decisions based on emotion – not logic.

B. Offering complimentary spinal exams for their family and friends with the opportunity to sign them up. The free exam offer only applies if they sign them up that night.

C. Have a specially prepared packet of information for the patients to pick up at the front desk. The D.C. giving the class should just mention in closing that they may obtain the packet at the front desk as they leave.

4) The C.A.'s Involvement

As the guests exit and stop at the C.A.'s station, he/she should say the following prior to handing them the packet of information: "And who are you going to sign up tonight?" No more and no less!!!

He/she would make any necessary appointments, then hand the guest/patient the packet of information. The idea is to not socialize but keep things moving while signing up potential new patients in the appointment book.

In summary, the spinal health care class offers stability and consistent growth in your practice. It takes the roller coaster effect out of the practice. While other practices suffer the effects of a shifting economy, the practice which utilizes spinal health care classes will continue to grow.

After personally discussing with nearly every chiropractor that runs a high-level practice, there is no question as to the importance of spinal health care class in their practices.

Let it rain and storm - we're prepared. My umbrella always stands ready.

THE PRICE OF INDIFFERENCE

One of the greatest causes for failure or mediocre growth

in all walks of life is indifference. And yet, as simple as it may seem to correct, more businesses suffer from this impersonal attitude than I care to talk about. It lurks in grocery stores, retail stores, clinics and businesses; it is even found in families – which is the greatest tragedy of all.

Possibly the following story will help clarify my point. I call it my Uncle Marty story.

Actually, Uncle Marty isn't my uncle, but the type of individual that everyone would love to have as an uncle. He is actually an uncle of one of my very close friends, John.

One night, Uncle Marty, John and I were discussing the value of confession. All of us being Catholics and going to confession regularly, we had some questions regarding confession and its value when there were no great sins to confess. "If I haven't killed, stolen, or committed any great acts of violence why should I go?" There was no question as to the sacrament as the church teaches it – only when and how severe the act must be before one goes.

At this point, Uncle Marty told us of his early life. It seems that he was going to be a priest and he went to the seminary to study as a young man. He further explained that he went to confession on a daily basis. Both John and I were a bit confused. Both of us wondered why anyone that lived in a very sheltered and devoted lifestyle would go to confession on a daily basis. However, it soon became clear to us, once he explained why. He said, "Boys, you don't understand. I didn't go to confess the sins of commission as much as the sins of omission. It's not what I did so much as what I failed to do." So, too, with our practices and patients.

It's not what you do as much as what you fail to do.

The two most common areas where you find indifference are: 1) with the treating doctors and their relationship with their patients, and 2) with the front desk C.A. This can occur because of the C.A. being under-supervised (train and leave them alone attitude) or the C.A. is being overworked by understaffing. Indifference can show anywhere at any time when people get off purpose.

WHY DO MOST PATIENTS QUIT A PRACTICE?

10% Move
1% Die
5% Choose someone closer
20% Are not happy with the care or the results are minimal
5% Miscellaneous
50-60% Indifference!

You can eliminate most indifference by trying always to give the baker's dozen when it comes to service, and the other way is to always, regardless of what you're doing, acknowledge everyone. Stop whatever you are doing and if you can't talk, say "Welcome" with your eyes and a smile. With those two things people wouldn't need to speak. This is especially critical at the front desk. Be tuned in and turned on when it comes to patient care.

You are where you are today because of what you failed to do yesterday.

KEYS TO EFFECTIVE PROCEDURES

Procedures are the key to an effective, smooth operation in all walks of life.

The three most important words in real estate are location, location, location. In chiropractic, the three most important words are control, control, control. That is not to be misconstrued as manipulation of people. Effective control is obtained by good procedures.

We constantly tell our clients to get procedure into their offices, but as a word of warning – don't let procedures get you. In other words, procedures are to make things easier for the clinic and staff as well as for the patients. Procedures, if done effectively, not dogmatically, will help break down barriers and smooth the road for patients to obtain maximum benefits from chiropractic. Procedures, when adhered to dogmatically, will build barriers and obstacles and will tend to drive people from clinics.

When you find a procedure working in one clinic and not in another, you'll find that most of the time it is not the procedure that's the problem. It's the individual utilizing it.

There is no magic in a procedure. It alone has no life. The magic is within the individual. He/she is the one that gives a procedure life and purpose. For example, you'll see this in multiple doctor practices. One doctor can go in with a patient and deliver a report of findings and the patient won't want to follow through with care. Another doctor arrives at the scene, talks with the patient, and the patient consents to care. One doctor completes the examination of a patient, explains the need for X-rays, and the patient refuses. Bring in another doctor and there are no problems. Not only with doctors, but what about C.A.s? One can't collect at the desk even with the dialogue memorized. Bring on another C.A. and he/she will get a favorable response from the patient. So, too, with recalls and other office procedures. Again, it is not just the procedure. The magic is within the person.

What is this magic? Why does one person seem to have it and the other doesn't?

I believe all people have the magic within them. However, it is lying dormant in some people. The magic I speak of is often referred to by Dr. James W. Parker of the Parker

School for Professional Success, as F.C.B. - Faith, Confidence and Belief.

As a child, you have a tremendous reservoir of F.C.B. in everything from Santa Claus to fairy godmothers. They can make anything happen with a mere wish or the act of asking. Then, as we mature in life, we find that there is no such thing. . . or at least that's what the "educated" individuals lead us to believe. Later, at some point in life, you discover the wisdom of the ages - that there really is a Santa Claus and that you are your own Santa Claus. At this point you find your life and your luck turn around. You find that luck is truly where preparation meets opportunity.

Affirmations such as, "What you see is what you get," "You can if you think you can," and "Why not?" take on new meaning. You truly are the captain of your own ship in the sea of life. At this point nothing, or no one, can hold you back. We often speak of this as being inner directed in a person with great vision. You see it truly does come from within. No one can give it to you.

Always remember that you are the magic that gives the procedure life and not the other way around.

STOP PRACTICING RELIEF CARE

A measure of a successful chiropractic practice is the number of patients returning on a once-a-month, twice-a-month basis, or whatever you consider to be maintenance. Those are the people that really know what chiropractic is all about.

If you're a D.C. who's just into relief, you are just like a medical doctor - you are committing the same sins that the medical doctor is committing - practicing relief care or medicine with an adjustment.

A good friend of mine, Dr. Jay Kaufman, runs a very high volume clinic in the East. One day I looked at Jay and asked how he did it. He said, "How do I do what?" "How do you get all those people in the clinic? What are you doing? What procedures do you use?"

We were in Dallas, Texas, sitting in a restaurant and I made the mistake of being seated next to him. Jay is like Tremendous Jones when he gets excited. Very physical, or at least this time he was. He turned and looked me in the eyes with a very serious look. I had no idea what was going to happen. When all of a sudden he lunged at me, grabbing me around the throat. Then he started choking me and all the while saying "If you believed in the subluxation like I believe in the subluxation – it's killing people and starving and depriving the body of its vital life force." I believe he was creating a subluxation. He was choking me so badly I don't think he realized it. I almost elbowed him because I couldn't breath, and my wife and people in the restaurant were at their feet ready to restrain him. Well, to say the least he made a point and I will never forget it. His belief system in chiropractic and in the innate or life force that controls the body is very strong. He knows and believes that this power heals the body. That life flows from above down, inside out, via the spine and nervous system. He knows that the person who exhibits no symptoms is not necessarily healthy, but rather they could be dying a slow death because of their vital life force being cut off or altered.

Symptoms are the last thing that show up in a disease process. He knew that the biggest problem with chiropractic is that it works but it works too well. As soon as the pain is gone, oftentimes so is the patient.

Frequently we explain pain to the patient in this manner: "Just imagine slamming your fingers in a car door. You have excruciating pain, but you're not going to die. And yet, some people have some forms of cancer and have no pain, but they are close to dying. Don't use pain or the lack of pain as a measurement of how healthy or sick you are." And in the same manner, doctors don't use pain as a measurement of how many visits will be needed to treat this patient. A patient in extreme pain and in a wheelchair doesn't necessarily require more visits than a headache case. Don't tell people to only come back when it hurts.

You simply must stop practicing relief care. That's not chiropractic, that's medicine. It's far better that people see a medical doctor if they only want Rolaids (or relief). But if it's a cure they want, you are the person for them.

How do we turn that around?

First, do not set up a treatment plan revolving around pain.

Next, get your patients committed to a next appointment time. Either the next day, week, month, or whatever they need. Get your patients in the appointment book. The only active patients you have are the ones with an appointment in the book. If you allow a patient to leave the clinic without an appointment you are cheating them and killing them slowly.

I realize that to some the word maintenance is a dirty word. Again, unnecessary care is intolerable. But if you check the individual and they are subluxation free, don't adjust them. Prevention is the key.

WEALTH - POVERTY

Someone once said to me, "I hope all your problems are

financial ones." I laughed at first, but later that day I got angry, and days later I forgot what was said. It's years later now and the words come back to me and I just smile. I realize that financial problems are far easier to deal with than medical, emotional, or family ones. But financial problems can be crippling as well.

Basically, there are only two types of financial fears. One, is not having enough. The other is worrying about the loss of it. So, you see both ends of the financial spectrum are affected - both the haves and the have-nots.

A large portion of any profession falls into the first category. They exist at a level of financial survival - living from month to month just making enough to cover the month's expenses. According to national surveys, a third of our population has no savings, another third saves only small amounts irregularly. These two-thirds fight for financial survival. The economy and rising costs constantly plague them. This would apply to most chiropractors.

We have often used the 80-10-10 rule in chiropractic, but now it can be reversed and used as 10-10-80 when it comes to financial independence versus dependence.

Out of the first 10 percent, tithe to your place of worship, charitable organizations, building funds for schools and the like. Out of the second 10 percent, pay yourself and save it. Open a wealth account and do not spend it on anything but investments. Boats and cars are not considered investments - only income generating ventures. And finally, live on the last 80 percent.

Sounds so simple, but yet less than a third of our population can manage this. Those of you who have read or heard this all before let me interject one additional thought that might pull it all together for you. If you cannot live on the remaining 80 percent, you are living out of your means and are out of your league. The key is to manage the income level you are at right now.

It is almost impossible to live a creative, fulfilled life with high self-esteem when you are worried about financial survival.

The second kind of fear is worrying about losing what we have. When it becomes an obsession it causes ulcers, constant fears and suspicion. This kills happiness, enthusiasm and dampens the spirit of all who associate with this individual.

SELF-FULFILLING PROPHECIES

It has been often said that what we fear most will eventually come to pass. Fear of poverty, however it manifests itself, develops due to a poverty consciousness and that consciousness will ensure that lifestyle.

Along that same thinking, those who fear losing what they have will end up losing much more than money. They usually lose their enjoyment of life as well.

Very few of us are immune to financial fears, but we must assess whether we control our circumstances or whether they control us. All of us need to improve our prosperity consciousness.

Now, here are a few action steps you can do to develop a greater prosperity consciousness.

One, make a list of your income and expenses (assets and liabilities) to see if your problem is, in fact, a problem or not. Secondly, if there is a problem, determine the amount of money it will take to solve your problem. Write it down on a card and program your mental computer that this sum of money is now flowing to you. Read the card several times a day. Always remember: you can if you think you can. What the mind can conceive and believe, it can achieve. Third, always speak of abundance and associate with people who speak of abundance. Gravitate toward those who have confidence in their ability to prosper regardless of economic conditions. Fourth, read positive self-help books, listen to tapes, always be on guard as to what is fed into your computer. Garbage in . . . garbage out. Be selective. Fifth, Q + Q + A = Compensation. What this means to you in your practice is: Quality plus Quantity plus Attitude will determine your prosperity.

Always understand that we all have different levels of prosperity-poverty consciousness – our own set of beliefs of what we deserve. This is all based on our past conditions and experiences. Our dominant thoughts will in time manifest themselves into physical reality. It truly can be said that prosperity or poverty is a state of mind. And since it is, it can be controlled and regulated for our benefit.

Another source of wealth has nothing to do with money. Rather than the accumulation of money, wealth can also be looked upon as knowledge, confidence and attitude.

Take away all my materialism, or what the world sees as wealth, but I'll always have what really counts . . . my own resources. My time. My ability to communicate. My courage. My knowledge. This can change your reality at any time and you don't have to spend any money to get success. It corresponds with autonomy, which is real wealth.

It has nothing to do with accumulation of money. It comes from knowing you can always change your strategies and come up to the top.

To be poor of pocketbook is only temporary, but to be poor in confidence and hope is true poverty and lasts a lifetime.

THE ACID TEST OF A GREAT ORGANIZATION

Most practices and organizations which move forward in the marketplace have sure-footed and goal-directed individuals leading the way. Their sureness is felt and becomes the lifeblood that runs through the veins of the organization - or in our case, a chiropractic practice. Their enthusiasm and continual optimistic attitude is the heart that drives the blood. So it is with a great leader.

But what happens when the leader is gone? What if something unforeseen happens? Will the organization survive or will it stop beating? This is a question that every leader (chiropractor) must ask himself/herself someday. You'll find this to be the case especially the higher your organization climbs and there is family to consider, as well as the livelihood of your staff.

This thinking may seem negative to some, but I feel it is a true sign of an exceptional leader. If you are constructing an organization/clinic of greatness, it will continue to thrive and grow long after you're gone. You may be gone, but never forgetten. This is because you didn't hold back anything. You trained your staff and doctors in the true principles of not only survival but continued growth.

A good example of this would be the Gonstead Clinic in Mt. Horeb, Wisconsin. Many years have passed since Dr. Gonstead passed away, but the Gonstead Clinic continues to thrive. So, too with our practices.

What was accomplished if it all goes when you do? Great leaders form great organizations with a great legacy.

If you were the last chiropractor in the world, would chiropractic survive?

WHAT CAN MANAGEMENT DO FOR ME?

"What can management do for me?"

It truly depends on what you need. You decide that, the rest is relatively easy.

There are many levels or planes of management and every person is an individual with different needs, wants, and desires. To some clients, the physical plane (procedures) of management breaks them out of their slump and sends them on their way. To others, to bring out the mental and spiritual sends them on their way.

Many of us at different points in our lives get confused and don't really know what direction to go. The greatest thing I could hope to achieve as a consultant is to bring out in an individual the belief system in themselves and get that individual to start dreaming their own impossible dream. If I can expose and show an individual his or her potential, then I have achieved a purpose.

A consultant serves as a teacher – we all have had many teachers in our lives, from academics, to parents, to everyday acquaintances. Most of us can only think of a few teachers that truly impressed us in our lifetimes, and yet when asked what it was that they taught us it's rare that we will be able to recall or put our finger on anything concrete. We remember the individuals and the examples they set, and how they made us feel about ourselves, along with the belief system they put in our own abilities. (Thanks, Charlie).

Each individual's need for management is different and truly unique only to themselves. For some it is procedures, for others it is a belief in the product (chiropractic) they are selling, and yet for others it is a belief in one's self.

DR. HANCZARYK'S SEVEN STEPS TO CHIROPRACTIC SUCCESS

1) Have an umbrella of protection by educating patients through a spinal care class.
2) Don't show an attitude of indifference, the number one reason patients leave you.
3) Install and use good procedures - the key but not the magic.
4) Don't practice relief care exclusively. . . this is medical practice with an adjustment.
5) Know and recognize true wealth.
6) Acknowledge the acid test of greatness - being happy with your practice life.
7) Invite - and respond to - constructive criticism.

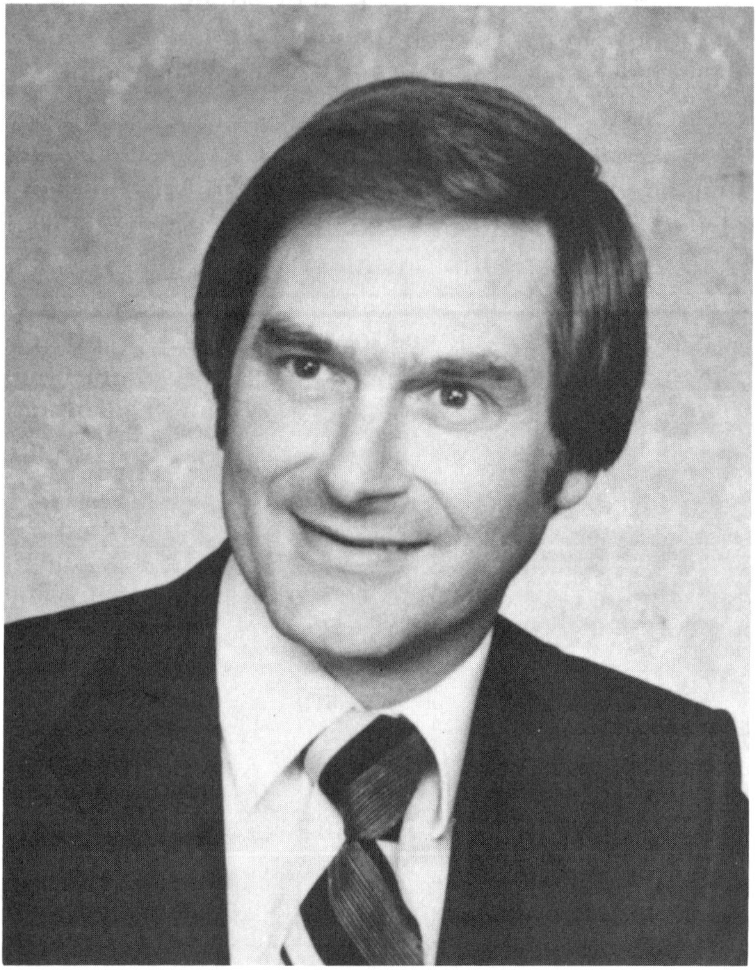

David J. Kats, D.C.

DAVID J. KATS, D.C.

KATS MANAGEMENT SERVICES

A dominant force in chiropractic management in the Midwest, David J. Kats, D.C., promotes and teaches his moral and ethical procedures to clients who wish to build a practice yet proliferate the professional image and standing of chiropractic.

His methods are "tried and true," demonstrated by the success of Kats Chiropractic Center, Lincoln, Nebraska, established in 1977.

Dr. Kats began teaching anatomy and physiology at Palmer College of Chiropractic, graduating Summa Cum Laude in 1976.

In addition to guiding his management clients to moral and ethical success, he is a team teacher at Parker Chiropractic Research Foundation.

In appreciation for his many contributions to the chiropractic profession, Dr. Kats has been honored with the Parker Chiropractor of the Year Award and the Outstanding Services Award of the Nebraska Chiropractic Physician's Association, as well as nomination for Nebraska Chiropractor of the Year.

KATS MANAGEMENT SERVICES
70th & Van Dorn, Lincoln, Nebraska 68506
(402) 483-7789 • (800) 835-7427, ext. 175

NOTES / GOALS:

CHAPTER 4
Goal Setting – The Racer's Edge

David J. Kats, D.C.

Goal setting, more than any other procedure, has allowed me to reach the top. That is not an ego statement, but a statement of thanks to the many people who have influenced and shaped my life. . . to those who have helped me understand the contents of this chapter.

AN AUTOBIOGRAPHY

When we hear of ultrasuccessful practices we tend to think that the doctors responsible for those practices must be some superhuman persons. Actually, that is not true.

Most ultrasuccessful practices are headed by doctors who know where they want to go, how to get there, and have the desire. . .other than these qualifications, they are very normal.

It has been said that the average American is not average unless he considers himself above average. I suppose that is about where I would place myself.

I grew up on a farm. We had a good, God-fearing family which provided the basis for strong growth concepts. As for grades, I was certainly no superstar. In fact, I have probably studied less than anyone who has ever graduated from an accredited college. My first semester GPA was a 2.4. A 2.0 is the minimum to stay in college. The second semester, I went out for football and, as a result, flunked chemistry, ending up with a 1.3 GPA. This placed me on scholastic probation, meaning if I did not get at least a 2.0 the following semester, I would not be allowed to come back to school.

The following semester, I got four C's and a D, giving me approximately a 1.8 grade average. I went to the instructor who gave me a D and pleaded with him until my grade was changed from a D to a C. It was a music course and the instructor told me he would change my grade if I promised to take at least one more music course in college. The next semester, I took a one-hour music course entitled "Chorus."

My study habits were actually worse than my grades. I never bought a book or took a note in college until the second semester of my junior year. I had an economics course with my girlfriend (now my wife, Diane) and I thought I would impress her by buying a book and taking notes! Don't laugh, it must have worked.

After graduation from college, I taught science in a small school for a few years and then went into professional music.

I sang in a gospel group as a full-time occupation doing mainly one-night stands in churches and auditoriums throughout the United States.

While on the road singing, I called home one night to

ask my wife if she had found a job. She related to me that she had two job opportunities - one to work for a chiropractor, and the other to work for the State of Nebraska. With the State, she would have a responsible position and would be able to drive a State car. I clearly remember saying to her just before I hung up, "The final decision is yours, Diane, but if I were you, I would think twice about working for a chiropractor."

When I came home, she had accepted the position as a chiropractic assistant. How fortunate to have a wife who thinks twice!

After another year and a half, our full-time singing seemed to come to a natural closing point. Our last concert was at the Nebraska State Fair. Coincidentally, the Nebraska Chiropractic Association was sponsoring a health booth. That day, Dr. Harold Jacot pulled me aside and convinced me I should go to chiropractic school.

After being a very poor college student and having a "less than successful" financial experience in singing, my self-image was not too high. Nothing makes you quite as cocky as a little success, and nothing lowers your self-image faster than a little mediocrity.

I decided to go home and casually mention to Diane that I was thinking about becoming a chiropractor. She had a very high opinion of chiropractic. If she laughed and thought it was funny, I too would laugh and play it for a joke. If she thought I was serious, I would be serious and would actually think about chiropractic school.

When I got home that night, I mentioned it to her and she thought it was a great idea. We talked about it for several hours. That evening, I drove through the night to Palmer College; stopped at a truck stop in Wolcott, Iowa; used the truckers' showers to shower and shave; put on a suit and drove the last few miles to Palmer College.

Forty minutes later I walked out as an enrolled student.

The requirements were not exactly overwhelming at the time! In fact, they were not even whelming! Although everyone should have an opportunity to become a chiropractor, I am glad that requirements have become so much more stringent.

The rest is basically history. I graduated from Palmer College with approximately a 3.9 average, went into practice in 1977 and sold my practice to retire into full-time management in 1984.

BASE HITS VS. HOME RUNS

Each doctor seems to be looking for the one key to success or those few steps necessary to have an ultrasuccessful practice. Unfortunately in chiropractic, as in any other profession, there are very few home runs. The successful practitioner is usually a person who gets one good, solid base hit after another. If there are any home runs in chiropractic, it would be the ability to set and reach goals.

A THOROUGH HOUSECLEANING

You can tell the size of a building by looking at the depth and the strength of its foundation. The same is true of a good practice.

If you are going to build a large practice that remains large and profitable, it is necessary to start with a good foundation. If you are already in practice, you may have to bolster your present foundation. This is accomplished by doing a thorough housecleaning – getting rid of unprofessional habits, bad ethics, outdated practices, and poor mental attitudes.

To build an ultrasuccessful practice you have to break unprofessional habits - habits of coming in late, habits of leaving early, habits of being unresponsive to the patients or not staying in present time consciousness, habits of sloppy adjusting techniques and other procedures that may hinder you professionally.

Unethical procedure also caps a practice, possibly not immediately, but eventually it caps the practice. An acquaintance was complaining that he could not sell his practice when he retired. He was actually skimming so much, his practice appeared unprofitable. What a "Catch 22!"

Rendering more service than is necessary to the patients and, of course, rendering less service than necessary (the poverty complex) are both a breach of ethics.

You are actually more concerned about the patient's money - or your money - than you are about the patient's health. This would appear to be inherently wrong based on the fact that you are a member of a health care profession.

Old habits, old education, old facilities and old equipment are all products of time. They are the result of standing still professionally while the world is moving on.

Before you can believe in yourself, you must position yourself closer to the leading edge of chiropractic. Improving your facilities and equipment or updating your education with new techniques and procedures is certainly no assurance of success, but keeping these old habits means you have a good chance of failure.

In 1980, we moved into a new chiropractic office. I somehow adopted the attitude that now I had the ultimate office and did not need to improve or replace. I was shattered two years later when one of my patients suggested that possibly we should have the carpet replaced because it was showing so much wear.

Our mental attitude is the last area that frequently needs housecleaning.

Some people can benefit from a triple bypass in their attitude department. We have a tendency to place previously imposed caps on our practice. An example of this struck me in 1973 at the Gonstead Seminars.

I was introduced to five doctors seated around the table, all of whom had $100,000 practices . . . needless to say, I was very much impressed. With today's inflation, however, a $100,000 practice is really only a survival practice. Many doctors still operate at that level and because they're living in the past, they think they have a good practice. We should realize a practice can never be static. It must always be growing.

Consider the experience of the Great Houdini who was known as the ultimate escape artist. He issued a challenge that if allowed to enter any prison in street clothes, he could escape within a half hour from that prison. This challenge was accepted by a government that had recently built a new, high-security prison.

The Great Houdini walked into the prison and began working on the locks. After laboring earnestly for a few minutes, he realized he could not hear the tumblers fall inside the lock. He started to sweat as he worked harder and harder. Mustering all his skill - which was awesome - he could not hear the tumblers fall, indicating the lock was opening. After working for over half an hour, he fell in exhaustion against the door he was working on. In astonishment, Houdini watched the door open itself . . . no one had remembered to lock it! This story is true.

For the Great Houdini, the door was locked tighter than any key could ever lock it. It was locked in his mind. Mentally, many of us duplicate this type of thinking in our practice. We believe we can only do so much. We believe doctors doing more are taking advantage of society, or giving less than adequate care. We refuse to admit they could do a good job.

To be fair to ourselves, we should realize we can do better . . . and cultivate a true desire for improvement.

Desire is mental. Desire is the force that turns the warm water of mediocrity into the steam of success. Desire helps us narrow down our goals and objectives and zero in on those things that are important to us. Desire overcomes fear and allows us to become creative. As you do your mental housecleaning, attempt to replace the fear of failure with the desire for success.

I've heard it said, "Don't let the negative few overrule the positive many." Actually, that saying is not true. A more accurate statement would be, "Don't let the negative many overrule those positive few."

RELEASE THE PAST AND REDUCE STRESS

For some of us, the fear of failure has become the reality of failure, and our practice has been less than successful.

We should realize, however, that at some time we have to make a fresh start. After we have done all we can to clean up our past, we must move forward. We should not carry past guilt. We are not the same person we used to be. The Bible says, "Behold all things and become new." Therefore, take counsel from the past, but move into the present.

Almost every week I am in contact with doctors who have filed bankruptcy, or who are $200,000-$300,000 behind in their income taxes.

Without question, they are burdened with stress and

cannot seem to cope. But at some point we have to release the past. We must move into the present if we are going to reduce stress from our practice. Regardless of where you have been and where you are now, you have the ability to move forward. The last freedom we lose is the freedom to dream within given parameters.

Reducing stress seems to be of the essence today. Classes are available to reduce physical stress, reduce mental stress, reduce emotional stress and remove spiritual stress. In fact, if you have any type of stress, you can find a class to deal with it.

Not all stress is bad. Some stress is exciting and can be a driving force. Deadlines, old achievements and previous past goals all give you certain amounts of stress that translate into excitement as you try to supercede those previous highs. Healthy stress motivates us. However, too much stress, unhealthy stress or distress leads to depression and lack of achievement.

Occasionally we can become overstressed and not realize why. Finding our stress, then, becomes a worthy objective. One of the easiest ways to reduce stress is to isolate those things that cause stress and eliminate them. Again, unethical practice procedures, poor procedures and outdated procedures all create stress. Living too close financially to the cutting edge or being continually behind can lead to stress. Deal with stress effectively by making a list of the things that are most stressful. Eliminate these one by one. The happiest doctor is the one who has stress without distress.

To find the source of almost all hidden stress, we must look inward. I had a client from Kansas who continually worried about being under an extreme amount of stress. First, he blamed his stress on his small facility, until he moved. Then, he blamed his stress on his poor staff, which he released. As his practice continued to waver, he blamed his stress on many other things until finally he was capable of taking an inward look and dealing with himself.

Most stress is self-created and most stress can be corrected if we are willing to take the proper steps.

STEPS TO REDUCE STRESS

There are three ways to deal with stress.

The first way is to give it away. Sounds simple enough, doesn't it? A client in the South listened to several real estate tapes. After listening to them, he involved himself in real estate far past his financial limit. As his real estate project started to crumble, the stress became evident in his practice. His practice drifted for a period of time then started to fall rapidly. As a last resort to save his practice and to escape total bankruptcy, the client allowed his real estate and his $400,000 of equity to be repossessed by the bank.

Was this a good move? In my opinion, it was. His practice is again growing and producing normally. He could have either lost the real estate, the $400,000 and his practice, or sacrificed the real estate and saved his practice because of a reduction of stress.

Sometimes we must take one step backward before we can take two forward. I had a piece of real estate a few years ago that was psychologically a drain on my practice. It moved from the area of healthy stress to a place of distress. During the Christmas season of last year, I gave it away to a Christian charitable organization. It made us both happy; they got a building and I got relief.

The second way to reduce stress is simply to deal with it. There is a direct relationship between the perplexity of a problem before you start it and the excitement that grips you immediately after the task is started. Occasionally, we must simply take the bull by the horns and deal with it. Getting started is half the battle.

The third way to reduce stress is to accept it. This may be the least desirable way, but it is still a viable alternative. Accept it and move on to bigger and better things.

REDUCE FINANCIAL STRESS

Frequently, we create undue stress by living too close to the cutting edge.

Each year the average American family continues to spend more than it earns. Practices grossing four or five hundred thousand dollars are going into bankruptcy. Chiropractors with some of the highest incomes in the U.S. are hopelessly in debt and stress-ridden. One of the major ways of reducing stress and increasing happiness is by maintaining a margin between your income and spending.

REDUCE STRESS TODAY

By reducing stress, you can be happy – right now, here, today.

Some people have so much stress they tend to live in the past. Some people have so much stress they tend to live in the future. But you can only be happy today. A person who lives in the past continues to talk about the good old times, the way things were before they allowed advertising, the way things were when there wasn't a chiropractor on every corner, the way things were when they taught you what you really needed to know in chiropractic college, the way things were back in the "good old days."

People who live in the future talk about how well they will do tomorrow, how "when they get rich" they're going to have a nice office, when they get rich they're going to buy new equipment, when they have a lot of patients they're going to hold spinal care classes. They relate all the things they are going to do when "their ship comes in." One thing you should be aware of, however, you should never expect your ship to come in if you never sent one out.

You can remember the happiness of the past and you can plan for happiness in the future, but you can only be happy today. Reduce excess stress and make your life happy again.

SET YOUR GOALS

This goal setting section is more academic, but still exciting. You see, goal setting is not something that you do occasionally. Goal setting is a way of life.

Step 1. **Make a list.**

The first step in goal setting is to make a list of all the things you want to have, do and become. This is your time to dream, not a time for calculated planning, but actually dreaming. What would you do if you knew you could not fail? Make a list of these things. Sit down today and write a list of everything that you really want. Usually we find people's lists vary between 15 and 25 items. These items will become your goals.

Step 2. **Arrange your goals in chronological order.**

Give the most important goal first priority. For example, if your most important goal is a new office building, make that number one on your list. Decide how soon you would like to have that new office building. Then, move to the second most important goal on your list and place a date behind that goal. Perhaps your second goal is to have an associate doctor. Place a date behind that goal and so on until you have a date behind each of the goals on your list.

Step 3. **Be specific with your goals.**

If a goal is to be accomplished, it must be specific. To say, "I would like to have a new office building sometime," is not a goal. To say, "I would like a new 3,000-square-foot office building with an all-brick exterior, done in oak trim for a total cost of less than $200,000, and I would like that building by December 31, 1990," is a goal. If you write that goal down, you then have a specific goal. We have to stop constructing wandering generalities and start contemplating meaningful specifics.

While at school in Palmer, I would make the 385-mile trip home to Lincoln, Nebraska, almost every weekend to carry on a business started before I went to school. I would travel home on Friday night, driving all night. The business would keep me up all Saturday, most of Saturday night, and all day Sunday. Sunday evening I would head back on the 385-mile trip to Davenport, Iowa.

Because I was exhausted from the weekend's work, I frequently did something that I would never do today. As I approached the interstate, I would carefully survey each hitchhiker along the side of the road. When I spotted one who appeared to be the type of person to have a driver's license, I would pick him up. In the conversation over the next half hour, I would ask the hitchhiker if he had a license. If he did, I would encourage him to drive while I laid in the back of my car and slept. One morning as we approached Davenport, I tried to convey upon my hitchhiker friend the excitement I had found in chiropractic. I tried to convince him he should know more about chiropractic, possibly even go to chiropractic school. I explained chiropractic to him with all the excitement I could muster, and said, "Wouldn't you like to do that some day?" With a very faraway look in his eyes he said, "Yeah, that'd probably be nice *sometime*." Will he ever become a chiropractor? Not until he changes his attitude. You can never get ahead being a wandering generality.

Step 4. **Create a plan.**

It is said that there is more than one way to skin a cat. Dr. Shuller says, "Count to ten and win." In essence, what these people are saying is that if you desire something badly enough, there is always a way to obtain it. Some ways are faster and some ways are easier, but sooner or later your plan can be accomplished.

Choose the best plan and get started immediately.

There are two ways to get to the top of an oak tree. You can climb the branches or you can sit on an acorn. The faster your plan, the more rapid your results. Recently, I talked to a chiropractor who was 52 years old and practicing full time. He told me his goal was to save $100,000 in ten years. When I asked him how long he had been practicing, he said since he was 30 years old. When I looked surprised, he relayed this story to me. He said he realized that to save $100,000 in ten years, he merely had to save $10,000 per year. This broke down into only $800 per month which broke down into less than $200 a week. When he realized how simple it was, he said he waited 22 years to get started saving. Don't let this happen to you. Set your goals and pursue them immediately.

Step 5. **Review your goals.**

After you have decided on your goals, set a date, and create a plan to obtain those goals. Write each of them in a handy notebook. Dedicate one page for each goal and review them at least three times a day. By reviewing your goals you promote positive thoughts. Use your imagination to visualize your life after obtaining these goals. Imagination is the preview of life's coming attractions - so run the movie.

Dennis Waitley calls this process self-simulation. See yourself having, doing and becoming what you want.

A recent goal of mine was to move into a new and larger house. As I sit here in our new house, I can actually see over 150 feet down a hallway to the other end of the house. The house has thousands of square feet, 9 bathrooms, secret passageways, gold and crystal chandeliers, a history including presidents, and more rooms than you can count.

It's exactly what I visualized. In my mind, I walked through the house so many times that I was afraid when they laid the new carpet, it would be worn from all the mental use. Review your goals each day and visualize them.

Step 6. **Do it now.**

Be your own boss and dictate your own lifestyle. Take the cap off. Don't allow your performance to be dictated by other people's beliefs. Just because others have always followed their predecessor does not mean you must.

> One day through the thickened woods
> a calf walked home as good calves should;
> but made a trail all bent askew,
> a crooked trail as calves all do.
> Since then, three hundred years have fled,
> and I infer the calf is dead.
> But still he left behind his trail;
> and thereby hangs a moral tale.
> The trail was taken up that day
> by an old brown dog that passed that way;
> and then a wise bellweather sheep
> pursued the trail o'er vale and steep

and drew the flock behind him, too,
as good bellweathers always do.
From that day, o'er hill and glade,
through those old woods a path was made.
And many men wound in and out,
and dodged and turned and bent about,
and uttered words of righteous wrath
because of such a crooked path.
But still they followed, do not laugh,
the first migrations of that calf.
The forest path became a lane
that bent and turned and turned again.
This crooked lane became a road,
where tired horses with their load
toiled on beneath the burning sun,
and traveled three full miles in one.
And thus a century and a half
they trod the footsteps of that calf.
The years passed on in swiftness fleet
and the road became a village street;
and then, before men were aware,
a busy city's thoroughfare.
And soon the central street
of this now renowned metropolis
and men two centuries and a half
trod in the footsteps of that calf;
a hundred thousand men were led
by one calf near three centuries dead.
For men are prone to go it blind
along the calf-paths of the mind
and work from sun to sun
to do what other men have done.
They follow in the beaten track
in and out and forth and back,

and still their crooked course pursue
to keep the path that others do.
They keep the path a sacred groove
along which all their lives they move.
And how the wise old wood gods laugh
who see them following a calf.

FIND YOUR ENJOYMENT IN LIFE

Unfortunately for many doctors, chiropractic becomes very mundane or routine and their interest in chiropractic fails. To be a successful practitioner, exactly the opposite must happen.

To be successful in a day-in/day-out routine like chiropractic, it is important that you fall in love with your profession. The most exciting workers are those people who have taken their hobbies and turned them into jobs. People who love to go to work are the most productive. (I recently talked to a client who had been involved in a rather instant marriage. He said the most exciting part of his life was realizing that he was starting to fall in love with his wife.)

To be happy in chiropractic, we have to make it our hobby. It has to become interesting again. That is what makes Kats Management Service such a successful practice-building tool. I treat it as a hobby. As a full-time hobby, to be sure, but one that I enjoy. If I could be involved with any profession in the world, I would do exactly what I am doing today.

MAKING A LIST

Do you really know what you enjoy in life? Most people do not. Most people want life to be enjoyable but never really spend any time doing what they enjoy. If you feel your life is a little bit dull or that you are not having fun, try this test and see if it brightens up your life.

Write down everything you enjoy doing in your life. You may be surprised at the little things in life that make you happy. Here is my list . . .

To play in the swimming pool with my little boys;
To spend quality time shopping with my wife;
To spend time talking goals with my wife;
To teach seminars;
To go to seminars;
To listen to good music and to create good music;
To do creative writing.

Hardly any of these require money (except shopping with my wife), but they do create happiness. Maybe the best things in life are free?

DO A LITTLE HAPPINESS EACH DAY

You can only be happy today. You can remember the happiness of the past and anticipate happiness in the future, but you can only be happy today. The reverse of this concept is also true. Not only should we do a little happiness each day, we should undo a little unhappiness each day.

Dr. Rick Rohrs and I set up practice within the same month in Lincoln, Nebraska. We became good friends. One of the things I remember vividly about our initial months in the office is we were both determined to build our practices by joining civic groups and organizations.

Quite by coincidence, we had both joined the same Jaycee group. The first Jaycee meeting that I attended I felt like a duck out of water. Guys were singing songs I did not know, smoking cigars I did not like, and talking business I did not understand. The only advantage of the whole evening was the fact that I got to stand up, give my name and where I practiced. Dr. Rohrs and I decided to attend the second meeting together. It was about 20 minutes to the meeting location and we walked in a little late. The room was filled with men our age having a good time, but this was not my lifestyle and I decided not to attend any more meetings. I glanced over at Rick and he was already looking at me. We turned around, walked out, and never went back. There are certain events in your life you can rid yourself of and, as a result, become happier.

One word of caution, however, do not stop doing those things that make your practice successful. Successful people are successful because they make a habit of doing what failures hate to do.

ENLARGE YOUR CIRCLE OF FRIENDS

Loneliness fosters depression. Man by nature is a social creature. Often we get so wrapped up in our work that we fail to find relationships outside the chiropractic office.

A recent study indicates that 30% of the adult female population in the US suffers from depression. That depression is most easily overcome by: 1) enlarging your circle of friends and 2) having definite goals in life. Study yourself. Are you the collaborative type? Most chiropractors are. No person is a rock. We all need support and friends.

CREATE YOUR OWN FUN

Dr. Mike Hanczaryk and I were recently giving a seminar in Denver. In the middle of the day, Dr. Tom Exum stopped in. He had been skiing over the weekend. We asked him if he had fun and he said it was great. He went on to tell us how he unintentionally went over a 50-foot embankment. Our meeting with him was only about ten minutes long, but he brightened our day. Late that night we ordered room service and sat down to relax looking back over the day. Dr. Hanczaryk commented, "If only everyone could be like Dr. Exum. He creates his own fun." And that is the key.

Happiness is an inside job. Recently, my wife and I vacationed in Acapulco. As we sat overlooking Acapulco Bay at sunset, we realized what a great opportunity we had and how much fun the vacation had been. The following day, we wandered over hills into a more rural area and found some little boys playing. They could not see Acapulco Bay and did not see the sun set. They were skinny from an apparent lack of nutrition, but they were playing in the dirt having loads of fun. Happiness is definitely an inside job.

A story is told about a mother and father who had two little boys who were very opposite. One was a perpetual pessimist; the other a perpetual optimist. They decided that unless the boys were more alike, they would have difficulty getting along together in life. So they tried to modify the personalities of each of the boys.

To make this happen, they went out and bought hundreds of new toys for the little pessimistic boy and placed them in his room. The optimistic boy's bedroom was filled three feet deep with horse manure and old straw. When the little boys came home, the parents told them there was something for them in their rooms.

Each of the little boys went up in his room and closed the door. Soon the parents could hear quite a commotion in each room. After a while, they went up into the pessimistic boy's room, opened the door and to their amazement realized that the little boy had taken a hammer and had broken every new toy. When they asked why, he said, "Ah, as I looked at the new toys I realized that pretty soon they would get old and dirty and they would stop working, the batteries would run down and parts would break, and I would be very disappointed. It would be like dying a slow death to see all my toys break one by one. I thought I'd just break them now and get it over with so I would not be so disappointed all my life."

The parents moved on to the next boy's room, opened the door and found the boy waist deep in horse manure and old straw. Straw and manure were flying all over the place. They stopped the little boy - covered head to toe with his new possessions - and asked what on earth he was doing. He looked up with a grin on his little face and said, "You can't fool me for one minute. With all this horse manure in here, I know you bought me a pony and he is in here somewhere!"

The moral? Create your own fun and realize when you have done it.

REKINDLE YOUR FIRST LOVE FOR CHIROPRACTIC

In the Bible, Paul exhorts the Christians because they have lost their first love for Christianity. This can happen in chiropractic, too.

Do you remember the years that you were in chiropractic college? Chiropractic was so exciting! You were caught up by the perfection needed to perform those techniques!

Do you remember your first years in chiropractic? The excitement you had when you got your first patient well! The excitement that was generated when you realized that you could treat almost any low back condition and make it better! The excitement you had when you realized you were finally breaking even and paying your own bills! What happens to this first love for chiropractic? Can it ever be rekindled?

Marriage counselors say that you can fall in love again if you treat your partner like you did when you first met. I believe you can fall back in love with chiropractic if you treat chiropractic like you did when you first met.

HOW TO REKINDLE YOUR FIRST LOVE

The first step in rekindling your love is to become professional again. Many of us lose our professional attitude. Our X-rays become less than adequate. Our adjusting techniques become more general and, in fact, sloppy. Our exam procedures become minimal and sometimes nonexistent. Move away from that trend and toward a trend of being more professional.

Second, avoid burnout. You have three choices in your professional life. You can work too hard and aimlessly and burn out. You can work at a good steady pace, grow and eventually wear out; or you can do nothing, complain about the past and the future, and rust out. I would prefer to leave chiropractic well worn but realizing that I had affected many people's lives.

The third step is to remove the ordinary. Avoid getting into a routine. Attempt to treat as many different problems as possible. Work either early or late, but not both. Share ideas and thoughts with another professional. Have a close friend in the chiropractic world. Create a brain-trust partner with another chiropractor. If necessary, form a partnership, a working relationship with another professional, but remove the ordinary.

Fourth, stay in present-time consciousness, Dr. Jim Parker so adequately covers present-time consciousness. If he could convince each doctor to stay in present-time consciousness with their patients all day, his mission would be accomplished. If we could constantly think about our patients getting well, each adjustment would become meaningful. Unfortunately, staying in present-time consciousness is difficult.

There are two ways to stay in present-time consciousness. The first way is to avoid outside distractions. Group your telephone calls and answer them at the end of the morning or the end of the day. Avoid handling any outside business deals during working hours. Real estate transactions, limited partnerships, stock markets and social events are fine and many times necessary, but they are not part of your business day and should be avoided until after office hours.

Recently my wife had occasion to be in a medical doctor's office. During her appointment the doctor received a phone call. When he answered the phone, he listened for only a few minutes and said, "Sir, I do not accept personal business calls during the day," and hung up. If we stay in present-time consciousness, it will revitalize our love for the profession.

The second way to stay in present-time consciousness is to visualize. Each time you make an adjustment, visualize the bone moving. Each time you touch a muscle, visualize the mechanics. Every time you use a heat-sensitive instrument, visualize the heat-generating potential beneath the skin. Concentrate on the patient's health.

KEEP ALL THINGS IN PERSPECTIVE

"For what doth it profit a man if he gain the whole world

and lose his own soul?"

Success is measured in different ways. For some people, success is a large practice, an efficient staff, getting almost everyone well, having a nice clinic, having a low overhead, having a low stress level, being financially sound - even rich. Still, I do not believe that people with the largest practices in the world can be totally happy if their stomachs are full of ulcers because of their fear that they may be audited by the IRS. I do not consider people successful if they have larger volumes of patients weekly than any other practitioner in the world, but their children won't talk to them because they have become workaholics and alienated family and friends. I do not consider people successful if they gain the whole world and lose their very own souls.

In our journey through success, we should make sure that we keep all portions of our lives in perspective. As a chain is only as strong as its weakest link, so our lives are only as strong as our weakest areas. Each area of our lives must be kept in perspective.

The spiritual, educational, mental, familial, social, financial and physical areas all need to be addressed. In your desire to obtain happiness, remember that even in today's money world, happiness does not go to the highest bidder but to the person who can provide it the best at home.

THE PRACTICE IN PERSPECTIVE

Last year, I visited over 60 different chiropractic practices. As a result I have found five basic types of practices. Properly categorized and with some work, a practice can become successful.

The first type of practice is a new practice.

The concerns of new practitioners are basically this:

"How can I get new patients in the front door; how can I get over my poverty complex; what procedures should I institute to ensure long-term patients; how long will it be before the practice becomes profitable; and, can I weather the potential starvation period that faces certain practitioners?"

The second type of practice is the plateaued practice.

This encompasses the largest single group of practitioners. The practice seems to be on one plane both financially and as far as patient volume is concerned. There are slight oscillations above and below normal, but the practice has levelled off. This usually happens when a practice moves from a physical to a mental practice, or from a mental to a spiritual practice, another concept handled well by Dr. Jim Parker. Quite frequently, it occurs when a practice reaches $100,000-$300,000 per year. However, a plateau can occur at any time in any practice.

The third type of practice is a stressed practice.

A stressed practice has a close relationship with both the plateaued practice and the finanacially troubled practice. Doctors in a stressed practice tend to suffer from boredom or burnout. The stress may be psychological, financial, physical, or a combination. Generally, the doctor has a greater fear of his stress than he has desire for growth.

The fourth is the financially troubled practice.

A financially troubled practice can be a new practice, but more commonly it is a practice in which the doctor and staff have overspent, a practice in which the doctor owes back taxes and has trouble with the IRS, or a practice in which the doctor has made unwise investments or has become overextended with excessive commitments in the business world. These financially troubled practices quite often have some of the best chiropractic practitioners in the world. However, to have a successful chiropractic practice you have to be: 1) a good health provider and 2) a good business person.

The fifth type is the associate practice.

It is one thing to build a successful single-doctor practice, but it takes an entirely different ability to manage a multi-doctor practice. The movement of a practitioner to a manager is very difficult. As a result, many doctors suffer defeat, at least temporarily, when trying to set up a multi-doctor office. Other doctors elect to stay in a solo practice all of their lives.

While multiple-doctor practices appear to be highly profitable, if established wrong, they can be eaten up by overhead and poor management. The enticements, however, of a multi-doctor practice - including semi-retirement, time off, and eventual sale of the practice - encourage many doctors to move toward the associate or multiple-doctor practice.

Locate your practice within these five areas. Possibly you fall within two or more of these five areas. Isolate your problems. Also, realize that other practitioners have the same problems. Realize that for every problem within your practice there is a solution that has already been exercised by thousands of other doctors throughout the world.

FINANCES IN PERSPECTIVE

I once saw a rather amusing statement that said, "Money isn't everything in life," and in small letters underneath it, it said, "but whatever is in the second place is a long way behind." That is, for many people, their concept in life. Actually, we have to keep wealth in perspective. Do not misunderstand me. I have been rich and I have been poor, and all things being equal, I prefer to be rich.

Probably the best thing you can do for the poor people is not be one of them. Money cannot buy happiness, but neither can poverty.

PHILOSOPHY ON WEALTH

You can have as much money as you want in life as long as you gain it through moral and ethical means, and by helping other people get what they want.

In fact, you can have all the money you want in life and not have too much money. But the minute the money starts getting you, that is when you have too much money.

Fortunately, in the few years I have been in the working field, I have been able to obtain a more-than-average amount of financial freedom, and while I enjoy the things this financial freedom brings, I maintain this position: If it were necessary to walk away from that financial freedom, I would be able to lay it down and never look back. As long as we maintain this perspective, we will have control of our financial lives.

LIFE IN PERSPECTIVE

More important than keeping our finances in perspective is keeping our lives in perspective.

One of the problems the average person has today is taking life too seriously. Approximately a year ago, I was arriving in the Lincoln airport. I had a tight schedule and had done a very foolish thing. I had packed my keys in my luggage which was checked on the plane. I was concerned because most of the luggage had already been unloaded and my bag was nowhere to be found. My concern turned into anxiety and I started pacing up and back before the conveyor belt, thinking about the terrible circumstance I was in. Just as I was reaching the peak of my unhappiness, I noticed a saying on a vacant billboard which read, "What were you worrying about last year at this time?"

Had my lugguge never shown up and had I never found my keys again, would it have been a major catastrophe? Absolutely not. Probably a year from then, I would not have remembered the day when I lost my luggage and my keys.

The most valuable asset to keep life in perspective is knowing the final score. Realize you have control of your life. I was impressed with Dr. Shuller's terminology when he talked about terminal diseases. He called them transitional diseases. If we know the final score and the final outcome in the game of life, it makes playing the game so much easier. It reduces the day-to-day stress and puts our lives in perspective.

In conclusion, success comes from an organized and well-rounded life, using goals to build that life and put all things in perspective.

Recently I watched a women's hundred-meter race. The winner, in a photo finish, won by one-hundredth of a second. The difference between a gold medal and a silver medal was just one-hundredth of a second. Trying a little bit harder, striving a little bit longer, seeing a goal a little more clearly. . . these conditions create winners. The race does not go to the swift or the strong, but sooner or later the race goes to those who keep trying.

Why leave your practice and your whole life to chance? Set your goals. You will grow. And remember, you can grow just as fast, climb just as high and be immeasurably more happy with moral and ethical procedures - and your growth will be real, not out of exchange with society.

DR. KATS'
SEVEN STEPS TO CHIROPRACTIC SUCCESS

1) Clean up any old, unprofessional, or less than ethical procedures in your office.
2) Release the past and reduce stress. Realize almost everything passes with time. By the way, what were you worried about a year ago today?
3) Set goals for your office and your life and spend time each day reviewing and reaching goals.
4) Find the things you enjoy in life. Make a list of those things and do them for a little while each day. You can only be happy today.
5) Rekindle your first love for chiropractic.
6) Keep all things in perspective. "For what doth it profit a man if he gains the whole world, but loses his soul?"
7) Educate your patients.

NOTES / GOALS:

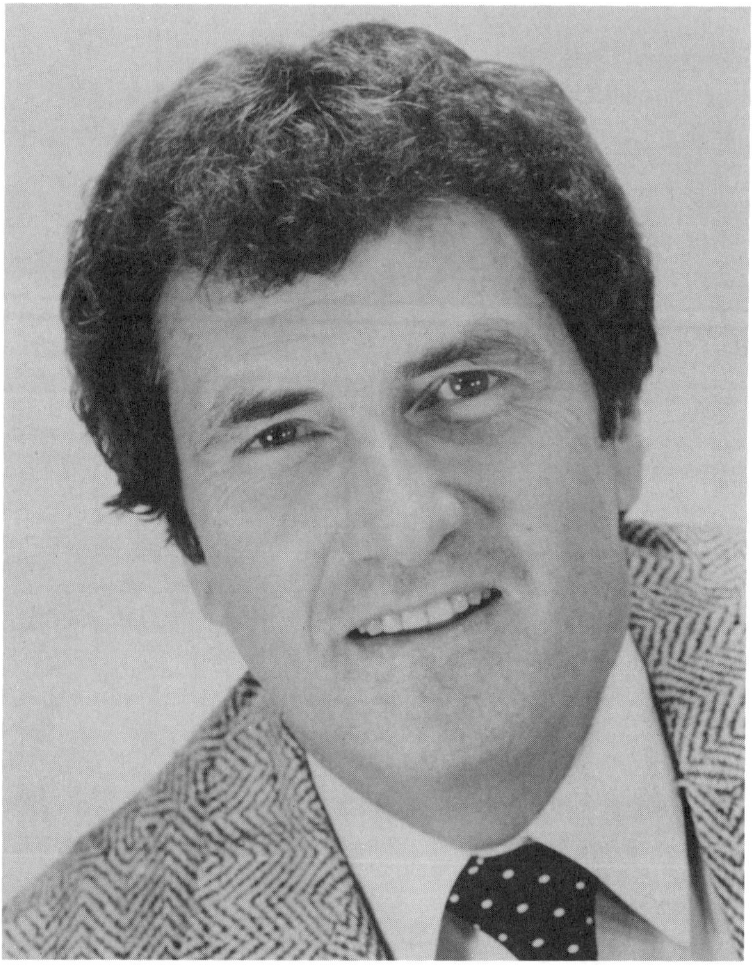

Lloyd E. Latch, D.C.

LLOYD LATCH, D.C.

LATCH MANAGEMENT SERVICES

"I've made all the mistakes in my 25 years of practice. If you want a large, multi-doctor practice like I have built, I can teach you how to do it and save you years of effort and several million dollars.

"My aim is to help you expand personally and professionally. I have assembled a team of 12 professionals to ensure that you get the care and attention you need so that you can achieve the goals you have set for yourself and your practice.

"I plan to put chiropractic on the map. Your expansion is an important part of that plan."

Dr. Lloyd Latch

NOTES / GOALS:

CHAPTER 5
Start a Fire in Your Life

Lloyd Latch, D.C.

I can't recall the exact point in time when I reached the conclusion that being a management consultant put me into the "What if?"-buster business.

I believe it was about the time I fully realized that nobody in life can be successful without a purpose. A person who says he or she doesn't have a goal or a purpose is a person who has a "failed purpose" – a purpose that met too much opposition, too many barriers, problems, etc. and thus failed (died).

A procrastinator is an expert at the "What if"/"Yes, but . . ." syndrome. This is a person who waits for his or her ship to come in, for luck to change, or who thinks, "Maybe something good will happen." This is a person who has put a "stop" on his or her life and growth.

For the person who fits the description above, I'd like to rekindle the flame and start a raging fire by offering alternatives to failure in this chapter of *Seven Steps to Chiropractic Success.*

I'd like to fan your potential fire, to get your original purpose alive again! This, in turn, will cause you to feel more alive and energetic! This energy, when channeled toward your goals, brings more life to your practice, and therefore, more growth, more health and a better understanding for all concerned.

Think of the beautiful feeling you had when you fell in love. Remember? Do you remember how you felt when the postman delivered your chiropractic license? You were in love with chiropractic then. Are you still experiencing those exhilarating sensations? Chances are they have wilted like yesterday's flowers. But – every one of them can be brought back to life again, to be fully utilized.

The way to accomplish this is to direct your attention back to your original purpose. Just review in your mind what you originally wanted to do or accomplish!

EVERYONE HAS PROBLEMS

Before you say how easy it is for me to say what I do because I've got it made, let me tell you one of my horror stories.

For years I'd been frustrated with having a huge-volume practice in a really gosh-awful building in downtown San Francisco. My daily wish was for a beautiful, new, comfortable and functional office building, a monument to our profession, if you wish to call it that.

Finally, things came to pass where Connie, my wife, and I were in a position to turn this ancient dream into reality. Call it Murphy's Law, if you wish, but about this time the economy went sour. Interest rates were rising faster than the Johnstown Flood. This was happening in the midst of critical negotiations for a building loan for our office building in the heart of San Francisco.

How was I going to pay 26% on a million-and-one-half-dollar loan? I had to be realistic about paying $45,000 to $50,000 monthly in mortgage payments for a new office. As a consequence, my dream began a slow fade, almost into oblivion. I experienced a "failed purpose" and almost - just almost - believed that it might be God's will for me to pass on the whole undertaking.

Fortunately, Connie persisted in tracking down mortgage bankers and other lenders in order to find financing we could afford. Then, out of the blue, a patient who was a loan officer for a large bank offered us a livable loan at one percent over prime and my purpose was rekindled. My fire had been relit. My dream became a reality.

Now, I recall how close I came to never experiencing the sensation of pride I feel when walking the corridors of my two-million-dollar office building, which reflects creditably upon the profession I love.

The point I'm making is, everybody has problems. Without a goal or a meaningful purpose, you're not going to go anywhere you really want to be. I've made all the mistakes in my 25 years of practice, but I've also learned from my errors. The purpose of this book is to provide a means to excite your interest in having specialists lend a hand in helping you get it all together in your office. . . and avoid some of the costly problems which can happen easily in every practice.

WHAT MANAGEMENT DOESN'T DO

Better than ask, "What does a management team do for me?" let's analyze what management doesn't do.

A management team doesn't set your goals or establish

your purpose. That's right. You must tell them what you want to accomplish personally and professionally.

Management does not solve all of your problems. Good management teaches skills and puts executive tools in your hands so that you can solve your own problems.

Management does not alter or change your technical procedures.

Management does not load you up with forms, scripts, "now I'm supposed to's" or other artificial means to run a chiropractic office.

WHAT MANAGEMENT DOES

Management helps you to accomplish your purpose, achieve your goals. They "light your fire." They assist you in directing the focus of your attention on the important things in your office: adjusting, supervising and leading.

Just as you believe in a holistic approach to health – we believe in fully helping you develop your physical, mental and spiritual approach to running and managing the practice.

Management trains you to communicate with your patients, your staff and your community.

Physically, you communicate with patients through your adjustments. Mentally, you communicate with your staff through procedural practices and by maintaining records and forms which make all the operations flow smoothly and orderly. You communicate with everyone in your community through your spiritual attitudes: the consistent outflow of thoughts and deeds which reflect your inner purpose to genuinely help people.

Where are your weaknesses? Management helps by locating areas which need change and improvement. Sometimes, the devil strikes at us where we're the strongest. You may feel your new patient acquisition program is the best around, but a third party appraisal may reveal some major faults, which, when corrected, could turn your office around completely. Discovering "blind spots" can be immensely satisfying for all those concerned. This is an "inside job" that must be worked at individually.

Every problem has a solution. . .your problems are not unique, but they can seem that way to you! Some problems have many possible answers. Good management helps you determine what is important and workable and what isn't. No one solution fits every practice. The secret is applying the right solution or procedure at the right time and stage of development of your practice. This is where good management can be of great benefit to you.

But, don't expect management to make you into something you're not. Management is not designed to do that. The goal of management is to get everyone working with a common purpose so your dreams can become reality. In essence, this comes down to procedures working in the office which have a common theme, a harmony of effort where the productive people get rewarded and the non-productive ones find positions elsewhere.

These are broad terms, to be sure. To be more specific, let's discuss the possibility of adding associates to your practice. This appears to be an inevitability in light of modern-day technology. The days of a solo practice are becoming very limited, in my opinion.

HOW TO HIRE ASSOCIATES

A new associate must be capable of demonstrating a strong ability to harmonize with the common purpose of the office. Money should not necessarily be the prime motivator – sharing the common purpose certainly should.

In our office, the purpose in hiring is to obtain staff members whose skills, work ethics and health philosophy mesh with and work toward our organization's goals and purposes. We want teammates who will help us win the game of helping others.

Replacing an employee in your practice can be an expensive, disruptive process. Not only must someone take the time to advertise for, screen, and then interview the applicants, someone must also train the newly hired employee. Until that person is fully trained and functioning, production will be negligible or at the expense of other organization functions. According to one study, this can cost you from $7,500 to $10,000 for an $850-per-month employee. It is therefore vital that this process be accomplished quickly and efficiently, and that the person hired be the right one for the job.

Hiring, whether precipitated through resignation, termination, or expansion of a thriving practice, can be a wonderful opportunity if done effectively. Hiring exactly the right people can help reduce resignations and terminations, and can assist your expansion. At Latch, So and Li Chiropractic Office, we have a staff of 32 persons. Our investment of time and effort into developing effective hiring, training and management procedures has allowed us to expand with minimal attention on personnel problems, and as a result, we have high morale and a productive, caring staff.

The biggest waste of time in recruiting is failing to specify exactly what you require of an applicant. Hundreds of calls from unqualified persons are no fun! When recruiting, don't use the office phone number in your ads as it may jam your phone lines and keep new patients from contacting you. Use another number (your home phone if absolutely necessary) and make sure there is someone there to take calls during business hours. Besides the usual employment agencies, recruit through college placement offices (business colleges, chiropractic colleges, etc.) and don't forget to put a sign in your reception area.

Start your screening process as soon as an applicant calls. Rate them on telephone voice, and call them back later to check their voice when they are not expecting a call from a prospective employer. When they come in, test them on the skills they will need if hired. Have the applicant take a typing test, compose a letter to a patient on a past-due balance, check handwriting for legibility; have an applicant for Associate Doctor mark a set of X-rays. Glean any data you can from the application itself. For example, how thorough is the applicant in filling out the form and answering the questions? Did the applicant follow the directions, are there gaps in the work history which might indicate a long period of unemployment or something the person wishes hidden? These questions, along with the usual employment history and education data, can give valuable insight as to an applicant's suitability. In screening, you are attempting to predict an applicant's value to your organization. The more data you have, and the better you use that data, the better your chance of selecting exactly the right person.

Once you've screened and selected the most promising applicants, interviews begin. Prepare both yourself and the applicant. Prepare yourself by reading the applicant's folder prior to the interview. Prepare the applicant by putting him or her at ease with your friendly relaxed manner and by mentioning something from the application. The candidate then knows that you were interested enough to read the application. Conduct the interview in a quiet place, free from interruptions. Ask questions which require more than a yes or no answer. Look for *willingness and trainability* as the most important qualities in an applicant. Get specific. Have the applicant tell you exactly what he or she did during an average day at a previous job. Ask about problems encountered at work and how they were solved. Ask what kinds of supervision they like best and why, what sort of jobs they do best, and why they want to work in a chiropractic office. Look, listen, probe and observe what is actually there or not there.

When you've isolated your superior applicants, check their references and make a selection fast! Superior applicants are in high demand and it is wise to ask them if they are interested in your job opening and if other job offers or interviews are pending. You've invested too much time already to lose your best applicant at this stage.

Once you've hired the best applicant, you're ready to begin training. Your new employee is still potentially valuable, and it's up to you to train him or her into a producing, fully contributing member of your team. Start the training with basic agreements. Tell the employee exactly what you need and want from them. Explain the purpose of the jobs they'll be performing. For example, the purpose of rescheduling a patient who has missed an appointment is to ensure that the patient follows through with the needed care and has the best opportunity for getting well. Have the employee read your office policies and procedures, then test for comprehension and understanding and clear up any questions or misunderstandings.

Right from the beginning keep a written record of employee evaluations or conferences between supervisor and employee. These will give you a written record of problem areas discussed (give a copy to the employee also) with the recommendations given. They provide a warning to the employee who needs improvement, and protect the organization from charges of whimsical or unjust treatment if the employee must be discharged. These records are also useful in noting commendations for superior accomplishment by the employee.

One of the most valuable tools you can use in managing your employees is to manage them by their production rather than their attitude, neatness, loyalty, or any one of a number of positive but vague criteria. Management by production is a complete subject in itself, but rather simple to learn. When practiced well, it will give you predictability, sanity, employees who are interested in their work, knowledge of who is really contributing, and control over the expansion of your practice.

Time spent in learning effective hiring and management of personnel is an investment in the future success of your practice. The goal is immensely worthwhile: a productive, organized, caring staff giving loving service to our chiropractic patients, expanding our ability to make sick people well, and assisting the healthy to remain so.

The reason for insisting the associate share our purpose is because cross-purposes can and do lead to disruption of the entire office. Since our ultimate goal is service to the community, disharmony drives people away from chiropractic, and that's not a representative standard of our profession.

MONITORING CREATES HARMONY

One of the "What if's" I'd like to "bust" is the concept that having prepared answers for common questions makes everyone into a robot. This is not the case with my staff.

Providing intelligent answers to questions patients frequently ask is just good common sense. The patient wants an understandable reply, which only an intelligent answer supplies. That's why we have new employees learn answers, so the patient needn't ever be in doubt.

A system must be monitored to be effective, and we do monitor office assistants until we feel they are both comfortable and convincing when giving answers.

Training and apprenticing is the keynote of this system, both for the office staff and the associate doctors. Practicing the fundamentals involved in handling and communicating with patients (actual drills) builds into the office confidence and certainty – intangibles that patients perceive and appreciate very much. And, when the patients are confident and certain about your office – they bring in many more referrals. This is most important to an expanding practice.

This concept of training and apprenticing with actual drills is an integral part of my management service. The value of it for doctors and staff is quite high – it fuels expansion of a practice much like high winds fuel a raging forest fire!

YOU AND THE PATIENT

Another "Yes, but . . ." I'd like to "bust" is the chiropractor/patient perspective some doctors adopt. Some doctors actually seem to be playing a role derived from their imaginary script of what a doctor "should be."

A successful doctor plays only one role, himself . . . and nobody can get a better part in any production than that!

Why? Because a doctor who has everything going for himself or herself understands that only truth and dedication are the constant factors, while playing various roles implies a wandering attitude, a diffusion of intent and purpose. When you're being yourself, the truth of your convictions is always in the forefront of your behavior, and it serves you through all the diversity of attitudes you confront with a patient in the adjusting room.

You come through with a truthful approach; you confront the problems of the patient and find solutions which he or she can accept.

I'm not implying some doctors practice dishonesty. I'm saying some chiropractors do not have – or have misplaced – the focus upon the force of chiropractic. Perhaps they are bored, thinking about something other than the immediate problem which brought the patient to their adjusting table.

Have you ever had patients who wouldn't let go of their problems? Perhaps they loved all the attention generated by their situation. And, have you ever thought that you might be imitating these patients by picking up their attitudes. . . by taking your problems into the adjusting room with you thinking your problems are also "special"?

Don't take your problems into the adjusting room; it won't make you a better doctor. Focusing on only the patient's problem will.

The late Dr. Gonstead taught me a gigantic lesson in this concept. We were talking in his office when I asked him how many patients he would see that day.

"Doctor, I have only one patient," he replied.

"What do you mean, Dr. Gonstead? There are thirty people out there waiting to see you."

"No, doctor, I have only one patient. . . the patient I am working with at the time."

This was a lesson in truthfulness and dedication for me. I learned that the power of this giant of a chiropractor came from a deep inner source of concentration which the patient recognized from the moment he walked into the room. Both Dr. Gonstead and the patient knew something was going to happen . . . and it always did!

It's not really important how long you take with a patient. What is important is relieving a patient's apprehension, correcting a subluxation and bringing a patient back to vibrant health. How long each visit lasts is relatively unimportant compared to the benefits you've accomplished.

How much is an adjustment worth? Perhaps this little story from my experience will provide a clue.

Some years ago I experienced a crippling accident to my hand. I went through the orthopedic routine of casting the hand and when gangrene set in, I went to a full body cast to receive the blood supply from the groin to the gangrenous hand.

I couldn't practice for six months and things were going downhill in a handcart, from 350 patients visits per week to 38. I was not only facing the prospect of being a one-handed chiropractor but a bankrupt one-handed chiropractor!

I'll never forget the belly full of anxiety I took to the orthopedic doctor each week when I would await his prognosis, which seemed more to me like a verdict of whether I faced a lifetime with chiropractic or a new career in law.

"Everything is coming along all right," he would say, and I would pay my $40 per visit with outright joy. The entire process took about one minute, but in that minute I learned I was still a chiropractor and that was worth much, much more than the $40 fee. Each visit I felt as though a 200-pound weight had been lifted from my shoulders. Speaking just that one-minute sentence brought me more relief than you can imagine.

If you've ever had a distressed back - and most chiropractors have - can you recall your apprehension? Your anxiety?

The point I want you to understand is this: when you walk into the adjusting room, the patient is looking to you for help. . . physically, mentally and spiritually. He or she wants your total power - your total interest in his or her problem.

If you are direct and your concentration is centered exclusively on the patient's problem, you will deliver the power needed to get the job done. What does it matter if all this is accomplished in one, two, three minutes or less? The important thing is to deliver the power of healing.

Going through what I liken to a soft-shoe routine which follows some erudite script and which takes thirty minutes to perform is not - in my opinion - the essence of chiropractic, or of getting the job done.

THE POWER OF CHIROPRACTIC

Management doesn't teach adjusting techniques. Your individual skill is something you must have, however you have acquired it.

Management develops your skills and abilities so that you are freer to unleash all your power in the adjusting room to get people well. . . without worrying about what's going on in the front, back or middle office. It enables you to be much more in control of your growth (predictable expansion) and consequently, your future.

To keep your focus on the adjusting room means all other functions are flowing with the identical enthusiasm you're putting out. This requires methodology compatible with your practice goals and objectives.

Of course, you need all these forms and statistics to chart your course and to determine if you're hitting the landmarks on target. Without some control, you've lost your rudder, compass and landmarks. . .you're sailing without a destination.

All these ingredients are necessary to build a quality practice equal to your potential.

Some of the confusion exists in the "What if?" concept which relates to the concept of practicing a "diversified" method. In this you apply whatever you have found most suitable from all the seminars you've attended in adjusting techniques. That's OK for trying to move the immovable, but it's not a solution for clear-cut office control. One program may "wipe out" the advantages of another system; they just won't interchange like adjusting procedures.

To flow smoothly, one concept is best. This is a direct course to practice simplicity, singleness of purpose and putting together an integrated team effort.

You learn to communicate on both a physical and spiritual level with your patients and your staff. Management is the science and art of bringing together many people from many backgrounds and instilling a common desire in these individuals to work toward a common goal of benefiting the health of the community.

Management monitors through specific systems on a day-to-day, month-to-month basis all the vital information an office needs to function without aggravation and stress to the doctor. In the final analysis, it's a method to free the doctor from housekeeping chores, freeing him or her to do what he or she does best, provide the best health services available in the community.

And that's the bottom line. . .a management service isn't just for the client, it's for the betterment of the community the office serves and for the betterment of chiropractic in its role of a health care provider.

Believing this as I do, I can say honestly that I believe this is a service worthy of consideration by every doctor of chiropractic. But, remember that having a management team in your corner is not like being shaken in a bag of flour, so everyone comes out looking alike, but, good management takes you where you want to go, helps you become what you want to be.

It's an "inside job" with each individual doctor. The key is personal attention. I've found this to be the one essential ingredient in building a successful practice. You can get all kinds of information from books, tapes, seminars, etc. The main factor is being able to implement it into your practice when you need it, and in a form that fits the way you practice.

At Latch Management we have built our program around personal service. Each client is given an individual expansion program tailor-made for his or her practice. The consultant guides each client through this program step by step, answering all questions and assisting with various problems as they arise. This truly is an "inside job."

DR. LATCH'S
SEVEN STEPS TO CHIROPRACTIC SUCCESS

1) Having and following a worthwhile purpose
2) Hard work
3) Attention to fundamentals
4) Top quality delivery
5) Rewarding production
6) Penalizing non-production
7) Cooperation with the team

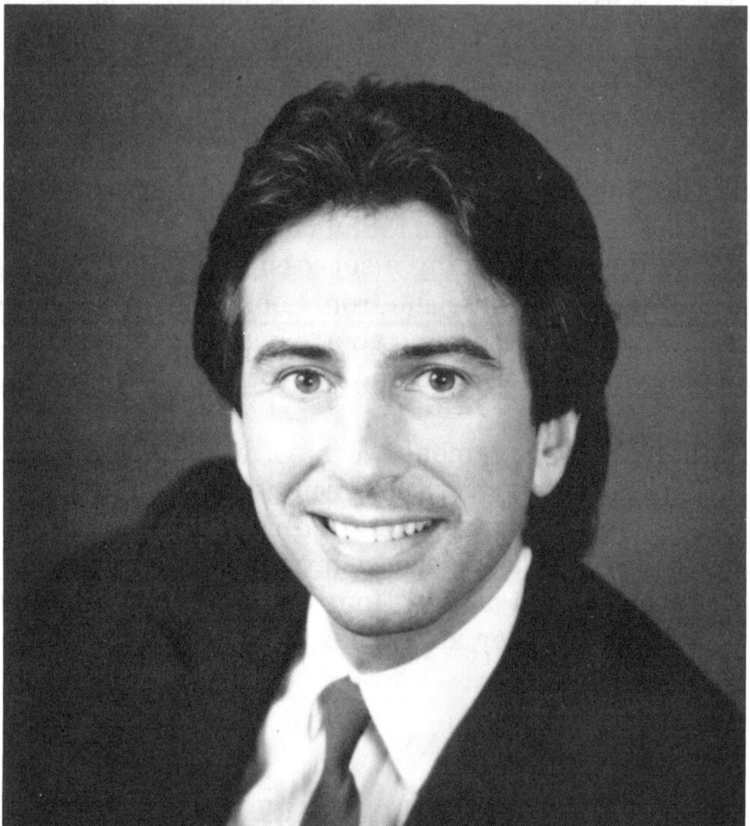

David Singer, D.C.

DAVID SINGER, D.C.

SINGER CONSULTANTS

David S. Singer, D.C., is founder and president of SINGER CONSULTANTS, the largest consulting program of its kind in the continental United States. His unique ideas, enthusiastic feelings, humor and ability to simplify the most complex subjects have made him one of the most sought-after speakers in America. Whenever he speaks, his audiences are filled to overflowing.

Besides being a management consultant, he has had a very successful chiropractic career. By the age of 25, his office was seeing over 100 patients per day. Within seven years of practice, he had mastered the ability to get new patients and averaged 150 new patients per month. By his eighth year in practice, his multi-doctor clinic was seeing between 1,000 and 1,200 visits per week in a state that prohibited advertising. Dr. Singer still helps run his office and, in conjunction with his partner, has opened two more successful offices in his home state.

As a teacher for Parker Seminars, he was chosen "Chiropractor of the Year" in 1976 due to his unselfish devotion to his profession. This unselfish devotion to see chiropractic as the leader in the healing arts has continued to motivate all that Dr. Singer does.

In his own words: "All chiropractors are members of my family and I own the responsibility of making sure they become as successful, happy and fulfilled as they would want to be."

SINGER CONSULTANTS
1001 Myrtle Ave., South Clearwater, Florida 33516
(800) 221-0385

NOTES / GOALS:

CHAPTER 6
The Singer Perspective
David Singer, D.C.

The most frequent question asked of a management consultant is: "How did you do it? How did you get where you are today?"

I'm going to assume that you, the reader, has this common interest of knowing how I got there . . . and I know of no easier way to answer this valid question than to start at the beginning – the end of my third year in practice . . .

GREAT COMPARED TO WHAT?

At this point I had accomplished more than most. Beginning in a small town of 18,000, my practice had grown to more than five hundred patient visits per week. Not bad, you might say, but you don't know the kicker . . . I was working with patients from 10:00 a.m. until 9:30 p.m., four days per week, plus a half-day on Saturday.

Planning and paperwork extracted another fifteen hours weekly in addition to patient lecture time. All in all, my life and practice had become the same thing. Here I was, deep in a rut. I saw no way out.

True, I had many material things that others thought made me better off than they. I could go to chiropractic meetings and slyly drop numbers to show everyone else that I was a "success."

So, why wasn't I happy? What was my problem? Everything I dreamed about through college was – on the surface – mine to enjoy.

Life was complicated. I endured a continuous loss of staff. There were emotional conflicts with people over money. I lacked the time and knowledge to create a tight machine. My profit margin was, at best, thirty-five percent. I had, basically, given up life in order to practice.

What did I have at this point? Three rewards: 1) Patients who got well, 2) Income and 3) The ego rush of being labeled "more successful."

The first reward was never enough. In a given day for every patient who said, "Thanks" – and really meant it – another blasted me and made me feel worthless. Money was great for the moment . . . like buying a Mercedes and feeling superior until it needed a tune-up, which cost more than my X-ray unit. Certainly, the ego rush of being so-called "bigger than life" never made me one friend . . . it, like the others, was an empty reward.

GETTING A PICTURE OF LIFE AT THE TOP?

That's the way it was. I was King of an empty Kingdom. One day, when it hit me real hard, I said, "That's it.

I quit." How can you quit when you're the boss? Who do you scream at? Who do you give the keys to and say: "Today is my last day"? There had to be a better way, but I couldn't imagine what it was.

So, I did what any rational, confused and confounded individual would do . . . I headed for the mountains. I sat and contemplated.

All the seminars and pep rallies that I had ever attended shot before my eyes. For no apparent reason a friend's face appeared in front of my eyes. I could see his face and hear his words. "David, you're young, have the energy to work harder, to see more people . . ." I lost my focus as I recalled this other "Big Guy" was gone from the practice scene after a nervous collapse. My thoughts drifted to the chiropractic Godfathers and Godmothers who had advised me and supported me over the first few years. Several had died of heart attacks in the prime of life.

"David," I said, "There just has to be a better way. There has got to be a different way."

THE FIRST REALIZATION

Let's start with the *First Realization.*

My goal in practice predicted my experience. My goal had been to see lots of people and make lots of money.

My new goal was: To practice without stress. To be happy and serve as many people as possible within the bounds of quality performance.

THE SECOND REALIZATION

So, now I had the goal . . . but no ideas of how to get there!

Every single method of practice I had tried had not shown me how to be free of stress, be happy, maintain quality and see lots of people. True, I could see only a few people a day and be free from stress, but that would deprive the masses of chiropractic care. Small practices seem to have their own brand of stresses which were economic in basis. Without a map to get there, I determined to find – or to create – a workable system by which my practice could become more sane . . . and I would reach my established goal.

Pause for a moment to allow emphasis on the importance of this Second Realization . . . I want it to sink deeply within your memory bank.

Your life is – like mine – a product of your primary goal. If you're dissatisfied to any degree with your life, think about your goal. Is it what you really want? Does it fully describe how you want it to be?

I recall sitting with a client and asking what his goal in life was. "It was," he said, "to see 'X' number of people per week." "No," I replied, "What do you want to do with your life?"

Practice is only a vehicle to drive you to your destination . . . it is not the destination itself. It is the means to an end, it is not The End.

"Do you really want to know what I wish I could do?" he asked. "I want to be able to travel at least one week per month, even a month at a time if I'm so inclined."

"For what purpose?" I asked. "To hunt and spend time in the mountains," he replied.

Although I don't count myself as a hunting enthusiast, my clients' interests come first. Therefore, I found great satisfaction in watching this client bring his true goals into perspective and eventual accomplishment. It's important to have the correct goal in order to achieve it. He reset his goal to have his practice increase and to be free to travel.

HOW WAS THIS DONE?

First, we wrote a plan and a time line. Within six months, his lifetime dream had become a reality. For one year, he traveled as he wished and only recently approached me to set some new goals and the plans necessary to turn them into reality.

Back to my story. . . I had no consultant available to draw a plan for me, but at least I succeeded in finding the correct goal. With this singular goal in mind, I decided to change all procedures until I discovered how to practice without stress.

THE BATTLE PLAN

Unfortunately, I had to go it on my own, but at least I had found the correct goal. With the goal in mind, I decided to continuously change all procedures until I discovered how to practice without stress. Once stress-free methods were in place, I would go after seeing more people while maintaining quality service. My happiness would be in the fact that I would have a practice, it wouldn't have me. Money would be available if I saw patients. . . and did quality work.

THE FIRST STEP

The first thing I changed was practice hours.

Every month for one year I changed my hours. I wanted

to find what felt best for me. I once figured out that the average patient spends no more than thirty hours in his/her lifetime with any given chiropractor. Yet, on the other hand, the chiropractor will spend the predominant amount of his/her life in the practice. Therefore, my hours should nurture me. When one is new in practice, it is appropriate to be available as much as possible. However, when one's practice becomes successful, the practice should fit one's needs.

I won't reveal my specific hours, but in essence I find I work best six hours straight and then end for the day. My clinic partner practices twelve hours each day, but only three days per week, on Tuesdays, Thursdays and Sundays.

In setting my hours, I realized I must schedule periods of time into my work for organizing and planning, as well as slots for meetings. Many doctors schedule patients for thirty-five hours, which I consider faulty planning since ten to twenty percent of the patient hours are required for organizational matters.

THE SECOND STEP

I had to control my time, not allow time to control me.

I started to plan my weeks and months in advance. I let go of being spontaneous to take control of time. The only vacation I took in my first years of practice was from sheer exhaustion and desperation! When I took control of time, I planned four-day vacations every other month and spiced these with several week-long happy sojourns.

With patients, I planned how many people I could see and how best to schedule them. The staff and I separated examination and report visits from treatment visits. Ultimately, we trained others to assist in many of the procedures, leaving me free to adjust . . . FREE! Free at last!

GOOD THINGS BEGIN TO HAPPEN

Patients started to fit into our schedule rather than the other way around.

When new in practice, I was available whenever anyone would see me. There once was a time I had an emergency patient on a Sunday. This patient now wanted all his future appointments on a Sunday. "Why not?" I thought. I would do whatever it takes.

I made house calls, store calls, apartment house calls, condo calls . . . anything to build my practice. My problem was, I had not matured to the point where I could take control of time.

To achieve my goal of practicing without stress, I analyzed what the primary stress points were. Later in practice I learned these stress points were the same for every chiropractor, but at the time I believed that I, alone, found it stressful to do Report of Findings, to constantly have to press for more patients and to deal with patients who failed to respond to treatment. Imagine how foolish I was to believe because a patient didn't respond – and the stress it imposed on me – that this was a unique problem! Nevertheless, I set out to confront these stress points and remove them permanently.

When I took control of patient management stress points, I found the time to handle the more difficult area of staff management stress points. More about this later.

The first stress point I confronted was getting new patients. What a source of stress it was for me. My emotions went up and down in proportion to the number of new patients scheduled on a given day. If ten were scheduled, I felt like Superman. If only two, I felt like Jimmy Olsen. I had become a board-certified YO-YO, up and down and loop-de-loop. Since my goal was clearly before me, I chose to handle this area once and for all.

I tried every method ever dreamed of to get new patients and observed several major truths regarding how to create a continuous flow of new patients.

FORMULA FOR NEW PATIENTS

The first new patient truth was this: To obtain new patients I had to be free of any doubt that I could help them.

This was rough because I hated to study. When I graduated, I celebrated that now I never would have to study again. Wrong, wrong, wrong! Graduation only gave me the right to go into the arena with the gladiators and lions. It did not mean I would survive. It meant only that I had the right to try.

MY DISCOVERY

I stumbled onto a lucky discovery. It was this: Anytime a person complained of a health problem, and I felt certain I could help them, they would see me.

What a change this was from my previous behavior. In the past when I met someone and I had doubts of helping them, they never came to see me.

This was a remarkable discovery. . . but it carried a price tag. It meant I had to study again! This was a fate worse than death. In years to come, I found there were two solutions to this problem. The first was to take as many technique courses as necessary to have total confidence. The other solution was to study the principle of chiropractic to the point of having certainty about the principle. . . and, with enough of this, a doctor's own technique will be employed with certainty. The key is certainty.

So, I found myself a student again. I took every technique course that interested me. I participated in programs designed to increase my certainty about chiropractic and my ability to help people. It wasn't long before I became certain I could help people. I read the original writings of B.J. Palmer and was inspired. Not long thereafter, I became certain I could help vast numbers of suffering people and even though I failed to help some, I was going to do a better job than most.

In essence, I became a healer. . . a person who possesses the inner knowledge that he/she has the ability to heal. At this point, true miracles began to happen and patients became easier to obtain.

ANOTHER DISCOVERY

The second truth regarding recruitment of new patients was: I could not be trusted personally to do the things necessary to obtain new patients.

This discovery was unpleasant, to be sure. But, it was a fact which I later found applies to the bulk of practitioners. There it was staring me in the face, I could only be trusted to press for new patients when my back was up against the wall. I hated selling myself. If I was a good doctor, people would find me. . .what a fallacy that statement is! Other thoughts I had were that patients seemed only to visit doctors who were in the public eye or who were more aggressive. This certainly was a stress point and the solution did not become apparent until the problem was correctly identified.

If I am thankful for one thing during the metamorphosis of my practice, it is that I clearly saw the problems. Many individuals blame, rather than examine, the facts. Others create solutions to either the wrong problems or to a problem which doesn't exist.

In the area of new patients, our most basic problem is our dislike for promotional activities. I gained some useful insight into this particular problem and found that it wasn't lunching with attorneys, public speaking, or any other of these promotional activities, but what I couldn't seem to tolerate was making the necessary routine arrangements to do them!

My talent was being wasted doing routine - although necessary - chores. What I needed was a good agent . . . There it was, like a bolt from the blue . . . it was so simple I could hardly believe it!

What I needed was a "front" man/woman to do my promotion for me. Of course, certain patients would boost me with referrals, but this was uncertain and inconsistent at best. The solution was a trained public relations staff member who would deal effectively with this vital area of practice.

I have never regretted this discovery and I question if any doctor can have a stress-free practice without the presence of this staff member. Although doctors inherently dislike being their own agents, they do love to perform the promotional functions and they do them well.

The agent's primary function is to attract new patients. They do this through making certain that referrals are accomplished, "Thank you" letters are mailed to patients who refer, newspaper releases are arranged and published, lectures are planned, meetings are arranged . . . in essence, the community discovers "Their Doctor."

THE THIRD TRUTH

The third truth regarding new patients reveals that new patients are a reflection of a doctor's ability to communicate. What one says, and what one means, are not always the same thing.

How you say something will do more to predict an outcome than why you say it. You can tell people they need care with the most honest of intentions. However, the statement: "You should come and see me!" puts people on the defensive, even if your desire is to help them. On the other hand, the question: "Would you like to come and see me?" allows people a choice and removes confrontation.

There is an art to communication and it should not be taken for granted.

The best public relation endeavors are useless without the doctor employing a high level of skilled communication.

I began to observe my communication skills and discovered I was a mess. I didn't communicate, I demanded. Presently, I have listened to numerous tapes by my clients - as well as observing their communication skills with people. Time after time, I witnessed how communication - the choice of words, the ability to listen, etc. - was so glaringly the doctor's principal problem in attracting new patients.

We all know a doctor who has no skill in treatment will not get results, despite the best of intentions. Similarly, the doctor cannot obtain new patients without communication skills. . . and that's the plain and simple truth. Another truth is, nobody said it would be easy. . . it takes practice and application, much like learning to play a musical instrument.

How about shortcuts to PR success, like newspaper ads? Newspaper and other media advertising is expensive and often attracts "shoppers," while PR effectively administered goes to your specified target area and is usually accomplished without a charge for the coverage.

Nothing can replace the results produced by a doctor who effectively communicates.

I have discovered an enormous amount of data regarding communication over the years. Here's the key:

No one came to see me as a patient unless, somewhere in the communication, they acknowledged a major health problem which interfered with their ability to live life the way they wanted.

My task, obviously, was how to get them to admit they had this particular problem. If I spoke with someone and they found I was a nice person, the conversation would do little to prompt them to visit me. On the other hand, if through the discussion they discovered they had this life-interfering problem, they then became candidates for my office. Let me make it clear, I do not condone manipulating communication to make people believe they have a problem when the facts do not warrant it. This not only is unethical. . . it rarely works! Additionally, it produces the same kind of stress we are striving to eliminate from our lives. . . and is contrary to achieving one's personal goals.

If a person discovers they have a problem, then you, the doctor, must inform them you have the ability to help them. This constructs the equation:

Problem plus available solution equals action.

A person with a problem who fails to recognize you as the solution might take action, but it will not involve you in the least.

The final part of communication is an invitation to participate, not a command or demand that they must participate. An invitation sounds like: "Would you like to come and see me?" We must be willing to allow people to say "Yes" or "No." True, "no" feels like, and is, rejection. However, if our goal is to reduce stress, we must invite people to participate and that requires offering them a choice.

HOW TO GET NEW PATIENTS

The basis for new patients is a triangle of certainty, reliability and communication.

The doctor who is confident he/she can help, will obtain all the new patients the office can handle, provided you use the required tools of a consistent new patient program which employs the level of communication skill required to insure success - and, you can have this without stress!

Once you establish a generous flow of new patients into your office, you must manage them and produce the results pre-implied. Many people think patient management is a simple process, others believe it requires memorization, others believe coercion is required. The bottom line is, patient management fails if it doesn't produce the results you and the patient want.

For years, patient management was a source of stress and frustration for me. It was a battle of wills to get people to follow through on their care. Every Report of Findings I gave was an attempt at persuasion . . . a constant stress source.

For sure, something wasn't right . . . but, what was it? Not that I wasn't effective at getting new patients to carry out my instructions, but my goal wasn't to get patients to do what I wanted . . . my goal was to be free of stress, and to have fun each day in my practice. The effort of convincing patients they needed care, must come back, and the other routine command lines produced stress . . . so, I decided to abandon every model of patient management I had heard of and start from scratch. I made a new beginning, and it worked!

Here's how the pieces fit together . . .

Prior to becoming a Practice Consultant, I had been exposed to only a single management method. After the first visit in which the patient was examined, X-rayed and sometimes adjusted, they would return the next day for a Report. During this report, I would explain the problems and resolutions, including time necessary for success. As far as I knew, this was the only model of patient control.

It should be mentioned that individual doctors have various goals for their patients. For some it is to relieve pain. For others it is to remove pain plus stabilize any and all vertebral subluxations. Across the line, nearly every doctor agrees that it would be best if patients returned on a preventative basis to insure constant good health.

One of my clients specializes in sports injuries. His patients want a quick fix. Generally, although successful, this doctor found his practice lacked satisfaction because his patients wanted relief only, they had no concept of prevention.

I asked him if he would like to have his patients on a preventative program and he said yes, but that his patients only wanted relief.

Another client did upper cervical work. He cleared out

patient's problems and corrected their subluxations within one month. All his instruments showed the patient clear of any nerve interference. He was very proud of his work, but his practice failed to grow. It was impossible to have growth when the average patient remained only a few visits. The doctor believed to have people return more frequently than his instruments indicated would be unethical. He was correct. However, the doctor did agree his patients would benefit from preventative care, but he insisted his patients only came to him when in pain.

Another case history involves two doctors who had the highest patient average I know of in the United States. Their average patient received over one-hundred-twenty visits in their chiropractic lifetime.

Each doctor practiced different techniques, but both were extremely specific about their adjustments and devoted a generous portion of their time testing for subluxations before adjusting the patient. When we understand the normal chiropractor sees his/her patients for an average of 10 to 20 visits, we can be impressed with the uniqueness of these two doctors. Also you should understand why I was so motivated to research their patient management procedures.

I was to discover during my months of experimentation with patient management that this field was incredibly different than I previously imagined.

My goal was to find a way to manage patients without personal stress, a method which created a satisfied patient who participated on a regular basis in chiropractic care. To do this, the first requirement was a willingness to change the way I had been doing things. I faced the risk of altering a program which had produced satisfactory patient results . . . to change now imposed a subconscious threat of uncertainty as to how successful I would be with patients in the future, plus the potential loss of patient volume. It was scary to contemplate.

The solution was - actually - simple!

I would experiment with new ideas on ten or twenty percent of my new patients. All others would be handled in the old way. This was a practical way to watch and observe what worked, the new cogs for the old wheel. I would create a workable system.

I recalled reading that medical doctors were totally unable to persuade patients to participate in any long-range treatment program. Approximately 50% of medical patients stop taking medication after one month. If medical doctors, who could strongly intimidate their patients with the dangers of non-compliance, had little result on a long-term basis, how could a chiropractor convince a patient they need preventative care?

Based on the medical evidence, I knew that any form of intimidation or a fear factor was ineffective and, of course, stressful.

I think it was when I took the Renaissance Program that I first realized human beings were able to make choices that best support them when given all the evidence. Prior to that realization, I thought most people were incapable of making good decisions. Thus, I would, for their own good, attempt to lead them into health care that I felt was the best. This made sense to me because if a child wanted to do something that would hurt them, I would, obviously, attempt to stop them and point out their mistakes. Although generalizations are not always appropriate, I couldn't stop recognizing the similarity between some children and patients in their attitudes and health care choices.

I am not certain as to how I came to the realization - due to multiple factors, I'm sure - it may have been an overwhelming preponderance of factors which individually held little meaning but jointly meant everything, but Pow! It hit me. . . I would stop convincing people what they needed. I would stop doing Report of Findings!

I would eliminate the stress of convincing people what they needed. . . stop trying to have people accept preventative care. Here's the reasoning behind this. . .

All traditional patient Reports held, as their objective, to give a patient a rationale for treatment. By this, I mean all that is wrong is explained and makes the treatment rational. The Report states what the doctor will do. Yet, no matter how rational the explanation, the results never were what I wanted and the whole procedure was loaded with stress.

SHIFTING GOALS

The transformation of patient management for me started with the goal shifting from giving patients a rational explanation of what was wrong and why they needed what I recommended, to the goal of getting them to have enough information to decide what they wanted for themselves. I knew if patients made their own choices, I would be free from stress. However, how could you get the average American to adequately understand enough about their health to make the correct choices? One must always remember that pharmaceutical companies spend ten million dollars daily to have Americans believe health is restored from the outside in, and that having no symptoms equates to good health. The "aspirin mentality" is no simple thing to oppose.

It soon became obvious that in one to two visits I would not be able to educate a patient to the degree necessary for them to make accurate decisions. After much trial and effort, we settled into a two-week long Report or educational format. At its conclusion the patient simply is asked, "What type of care would you like us to provide you?" Presently, approximately 90% of our patients choose corrective care leading to preventative care. How? Why? Here's the explanation.

PATIENT EDUCATION

Educating the patient was the first objective.

To do this, I tried everything, slide presentations, video movies, lectures and books. It seemed I was successful only at converting the already converted. Those who were not already committed to health as their first priority and a natural methodology as their vehicle were not influenced by my efforts.

The flaw in my system was trying to pull off the entire education within two or three visits. With the patient being told on the second visit what they needed, I tried to have most of their education done at that point. This action was not successful.

The solution was to begin treatment on the second visit, but postpone the recommendation until I was satisfied they comprehended what I wanted them to know. In other words, patients would begin their treatment, understanding I could help them, but uncertain as to how long it would take or why chiropractic worked. However, spreading out the Report made the educational process easier.

Nevertheless, I still noticed a lot of people would object to being educated. "Just tell me what's wrong . . . and fix it." How do you break through that rigid mentality? Out of observation, I eventually discovered the secret to getting a patient receptive to education and to my somewhat radical procedures.

A SIMPLE SECRET

The secret was so simple.

Give them the choice as to how they wanted to be managed! This is to say I would let them choose to be educated or not. Thus, my second visit served to explain to patients how I could manage them rather than explaining their health problems. In the Report, we would discuss if they wanted to be told what they needed, or if they wanted to be educated so they could make their own choice. If you give a person a choice as to how they can be treated, a surprising number choose to be educated instead of "tell me what's wrong and fix it."

Those who wanted me to tell them what I found and what they should do, I simply gave a standard rationale of treatment and my recommendation of care. Those who wanted to be educated and make their own choices, we proceeded to handle in this new way. Those patients who wanted the education would be scheduled for video programs and extended visits over a period of at least five visits. During this time, they would gain understanding as to how chiropractic works. They would discover the difference between relief of symptoms and correcting the cause of their problems. Once they clearly understood how an irritated nerve caused a loss of function, they would be ready to see their X-rays. The X-rays, explained from a chiropractic viewpoint, could be understood within our context because of the education they had received. I would also go over any other tests and results. On a subsequent visit, they would be asked to decide between relief or corrective care. A flow chart as to how this procedure would look is as follows:

Visit 1
New Patient Examination

Visit 2
Brief Explanation of Patient's Problem
Explanation of Types of Patient Management
Patient Chooses Management Method
Explanation of an Adjustment
Brief Explanation of Finance
First Adjustment Given

Visit 3

Educate Me So I Can Make My Own Choice

Adjustment
Explain how symptoms are the end result of body dysfunction and being free from symptoms does not mean one is well.

Visit 4
Chiropractic Adjustment
Explain that the body heals itself when normal function is available. The goal of returning the body to normal function is not simply removing symptoms explained.

Just Tell Me What's Wrong and Fix It

Rationale for Treatment
Test Results and X-Rays Analyzed
Need for Care Explained
Treatment Recommendation
Second Adjustment Given

ALL SUBSEQUENT VISITS ARE BASICALLY ADJUSTMENTS

Fig. 1

Visit 5

Educate Me So I Can Make My Own Choice

Chiropractic Adjustment
Explain the difference between relief and corrective care.
Explain subluxation or spinal adjustment's relationship to correction.

Visit 6

Chiropractic Adjustment
Review tests and X-ray findings.

Visit 7

Chiropractic Adjustment
Review tests and X-ray findings.

Just Tell Me What's Wrong and Fix It

ALL SUBSEQUENT VISTS ARE BASICALLY ADJUSTMENTS

Fig. 2

A STEP-BY-STEP PROGRAM

The advantages of an open, educational patient management system are many. The doctor need only leave five minutes extra per visit to explain one major point. Because there is only one major point to cover, the doctor can take his/her time and really drive the point home. If the patient misses the appointment, there is not a major loss of the doctor's time. Most important of all, a person learns better step-by-step and really comprehends what is said. The step-by-step method places the review of X-rays where it belongs, after the understanding of spinal and neurological dysfunction. Thus, the doctor can explain X-rays or test results knowing the patient understands the chiropractic viewpoint.

Because the doctor has as many visits as necessary to educate the patient, he/she has greater flexibility. Whereas, if the doctor tries to explain everything in one thirty-minute visit, he/she is forced to explain everything without flexibility. Some people can fully grasp what we are about and be made aware of their related health needs in three five-minute explanations. Some people require a lot more explanation. The doctor has the option to move the patient management at a pace set by each individual patient.

Imagine trying to explain to someone what chiropractic is, what their tests revealed, what their X-rays showed, how long their care will take, why they need to come in so often, what an adjustment is, how the finances will be handled, etc., etc., all in one visit! No wonder, when surveying chiropractors, the second most stressful experience is having to give a Report to the patient. It is usually so stressful because of the pressure on the doctor to cover so many subjects in such a short time . . . not to mention the hovering specter of rejection.

ELIMINATE STRESS

An open educational patient management system removes all these sources of stress.

Because this system is so radical, we recommend to our clients not even to try it until they have heard my explanation several times. However, if readers wish to experiment, do this: Examine what you want your patients to understand in regard to the care you offer. . . then determine the major points necessary to transmit complete understanding of what you do offer. The following step requires taking no longer than five minutes to explain each point to the patient. Try a "test run" on several non-patients - the staff or family members. . . if it works, try it on one new patient. Utilize the feedback from non-patient sources and if it works smoothly, incorporate this procedure in your daily practice and watch the stress disappear from your life.

There is one final consideration of patient management . . . it doesn't end once a patient says "yes" to care. Each visit must put emphasis on the doctor's goal for the patient, or the patient will aim their care towards their own goal. Since patients have one goal - and one goal only - to get rid of their pain/problem, we must reinforce our goal for the patient. As doctors, what is our goal? This you must decide.

My goal is two-fold, remove symptoms and the structural causation. Therefore, on each visit, I reinforce the concept of correction to remind the patient of this goal. You can do this with instrumentation or with specific technique . . . whichever method you use, make certain to demonstrate the need for care. The point remains that patient management is a visit-to-visit process.

THE NON-RESPONSIVE PATIENT

I used to feel guilty when a patient failed to respond. I would apologize and ask to be forgiven. I was just like my client in Massachusetts who, when a patient said he felt worse, proceeded to treat the patient for two entire months – for free! Of course, this was the subject of a lively discussion!

Here's the bottom line on patients who fail to respond: They need discipline, and they need to be placed on a stringent program of self-care. Instruct them that should they fail to show improvement with your methods they will be dismissed or referred out.

The reasoning behind this is simple. This patient oftentimes is a victim, and your sympathy makes you a victim as well. When that occurs, you and I have become victims of the patient's personal problem. You should understand that sympathy leads to acquiring someone else's problems. Empathy is understanding a person's problems/feelings. I stopped being sympathetic and became empathetic . . . much to my relief and to the patient's benefit.

With discipline, such as exercises, increased frequency of visits, etc., plus the knowledge I would reject them if they failed to respond, the majority of my patients improved dramatically.

Trust me, patients who fail to respond should either shape up or ship out. To do otherwise is sheer disaster from a professional point of view . . . you'll drain your time and energy, and it will contribute an enormous amount of stress. Try substituting discipline for guilt . . . it's a surefire remedy.

Now it's time to turn our attention toward the working heart of our practice – the staff.

THE THIRD REALIZATION

Earlier I mentioned I had three realizations. This is the third . . . it relates to our staff, without whom we cannot expect to function successfully.

I recall early days in practice. Each employee represented another potential source of upset. I remember hiring over forty different CAs within my first two years of practice. They came and went in speedy procession . . . to the point I was seeing more CAs than patients! Certainly, I hadn't gained control of this area and it was an absolute source of stress.

I cringe when I recall arguments over money, vacations, hours, staying late, going to seminars, etc., etc. Once I dreamed of designing a computer which would replace my staff! Each patient would have an identification card they would plug into the computer upon entering the office. Each adjusting room would be equipped with a terminal and I would enter the treatment rendered and the patient would be billed automatically and pay by mail. I would practice without any staff!

Obviously, my computer dream was my escape from staff problems for which I had no solutions.

What I was searching for through fantasy actually came to me through the realization that a properly trained and managed staff was the ultimate answer to practice happiness, freedom and relief from stress.

This realization was the admission my employees turned out bad because I did not know how to create good ones. It was like baking a cake and using all the wrong ingredients. In the end, the cake was not a cake but a round chocolate-covered rock. Well, if one bakes enough rocks it occurs there are no good cakes. Also, one concurs that anyone else who says they have good cakes is a liar.

The turning point in this area came, once again, as the

end result of an accumulation of factors.

I was so tired of dealing with staff upsets that I was willing to do anything, including recognizing that I was the major problem. It wasn't that I was a bad person, but rather that I was ignorant. Just as I needed to learn more treatment technique, I needed more management technique. Fortunately for me, about this time I was introduced to L. Ron Hubbard's book, *The Problems of Work,* which described my dilemma perfectly.

Apparently, when I decided I disliked studying, I also decided I disliked teaching or training . . . and, what a price I paid for this low-grade attitude.

The major problem surrounding my staff centered on the fact it was, basically, untrained. It was a group of individuals, each struggling toward their individual goals and survival. I was to find that to change a mob, or a mass of people, into a team was my first and foremost purpose . . . and at one time I found a hundred reasons why I was incapable of instilling purpose within my staff.

I thought they wouldn't be interested; I was afraid they would reject the entire concept . . . and in my sublimation I surmised, "Who am I to be preaching a noble cause?" We need work, I believed, not purpose. How foolish I was to accept these inferior notions!

However, from the moment I stood up and declared a purpose for our office, it was like the parting of the sea . . . a miracle of about-face. All gossiping fell into silence, rumors and accusations fell away and the power of purpose touched our office . . . like we were born again.

PURPOSE BEGETS DIRECTION

With a purpose we had direction. We started to move from being a mob to working as a team.

Here we were, running down field, with me yelling, "Go team, Go!" I was the quarterback, like it or not. The rest of my "players" now had the desire to win. They wanted to accomplish our purpose. The problem was none of them knew how to play their respective positions and I wasn't sure what positions were necessary or how best to play them.

Because of our lack of training and not filling all the positions on our team, we lost a lot of games. Many players quit out of a sense of frustration, they felt they were getting nowhere. If the truth be known, they weren't getting anywhere. . . actually none of us were.

After studying more of L. Ron Hubbard's management methods, it became clear there was a technology for adequately training staff and also there was a proper design to a successful organization. I found that numerous players who were necessary to make our plan function were missing from our team. I had been trying to play "football" without a fullback or a wide-receiver. No wonder winning was so difficult and elusive.

STAFF YOUR TEAM TO WIN

Learning this, I set out to train our staff and to have all the players necessary to play the game. We now have our fullback (a public relations person), our left wide-receiver (person in charge of products) and a right wide-receiver (person in charge of correction and training). . . and we are winning! Since all our players know their positions and can rely upon me to maintain our purpose, nothing should keep us from our winning pattern.

QUANTUM LEAPS

I often coach my clients in the first quantum leap – from "no patients" to "all the patients the doctor can treat."

The second quantum leap begins when you enter a multiple doctor organization, a sole doctor with numerous staff support in the area of patient treatment. Only a handful of doctors have been successful at delegating the majority of patient examination and partial treatment to other staff members who are not licensed as doctors.

The reason a doctor can treat only a certain number of people is due to physical, mental or spiritual causes. Limiting physical causes are: inadequate treatment space, staff, energy, etc. Mental limitations are: fear of burnout, the worry of how to handle a large caseload, being sympathetic rather than empathetic, unknowledgeable as to mechanics of efficiency, etc. The spiritual reason a doctor can see only a given number of patients is an unwritten personal law which states: "Everyone must do complete work."

From the moment the doctor and staff feel unable to do complete work they inherently reduce the size of their enterprise – thereby generating conditions which limit the size of their practice to the degree they feel capable of handling.

A person with high ethics never sacrifices the patient's needs for the doctor's greed. Like in a bathtub when the volume of water becomes too high, the safety run-off valve is there to drain out the excess water. Some doctors see only one hundred people per week while others see upward of four hundred. The determining factor on a spiritual level as to the practice size will depend upon their level of personal "safety run-off valve."

INSTALL YOUR MAXIMUM SAFETY VALVE

The way a person raises where his/her safety valve sits is through a process known as delegation and training. First, the doctor may delegate examinations, X-ray or consultations. Ultimately, the doctor can delegate patient reports, even treatment itself.

In the first quantum leap the game is, "How big can I become?" In the second quantum leap the game is, "How much can I support others to become big?"

The rules which make one successful in the first quantum are not capable of making one successful in the second quantum, which has its own rules and procedures which must be learned or the doctor will find he/she has created a monster. . . their practice will have them, rather than the other way around.

In life and in practice, as one moves forward the major upsets we face are created when we are stopped. As long as things are expanding, we generally are excited, even enthusiastic. It is this reason the name of the game is "Keep Moving!" toward a purpose. It's easy to become depressed - burned out - or to lose interest in your career when the feeling is you are getting nowhere. Trust me, the solution to boredom, apathy or lack of motivation has its roots in the further understanding of the game you are in and how to win it.

PACE YOURSELF TO SUCCESS

Bigger is not always better. However, when things get better they seem to naturally get bigger.

As I progressed from a know-it-all who knew nothing to a person who is a continuously learning student, I relaxed somewhat. Our practice is truly a vehicle we drive through our lifetime. It is not the goal of life. It is a vehicle for you and for me to express our life. To get to your life's destination, the better the vehicle, the easier it will be to get there. Just as our auto needs a tune-up and maintenance, so do our practices. Some of us might even need a new engine or some major exterior repair.

Someone said that when you find the truth, knowledge or, in essence, that which works, it leaves you only one thing to do . . . share it with others. As a result, I have dedicated my life to helping my fellow chiropractors to expand their practices, fulfill their purposes and improve the quality of their lives, as well as the lives of their patients.

I hope when I die someone will write on my gravestone: "ALL USED UP."

DR. SINGER'S SEVEN STEPS TO CHIROPRACTIC SUCCESS

1) If you don't like your circumstances, re-examine the wording of your principal goal.
2) To get new patients, free yourself of any doubt you can help them.
3) To have a continuous number of new patients, someone other than the doctor must be accountable to create those projects to bring patients in.
4) To manage patients successfully requires educating them. The doctor's job is to create an educational process that works for patients.
5) Staff is a problem if each individual is not adequately trained. A properly trained staff creates solutions and freedom for the doctor. The doctor's job is to make sure the staff is very well trained.
6) To continue to expand, one must delegate. Trying to do everything oneself is a guarantee one will remain small.
7) Maintain an attitude of confidence.

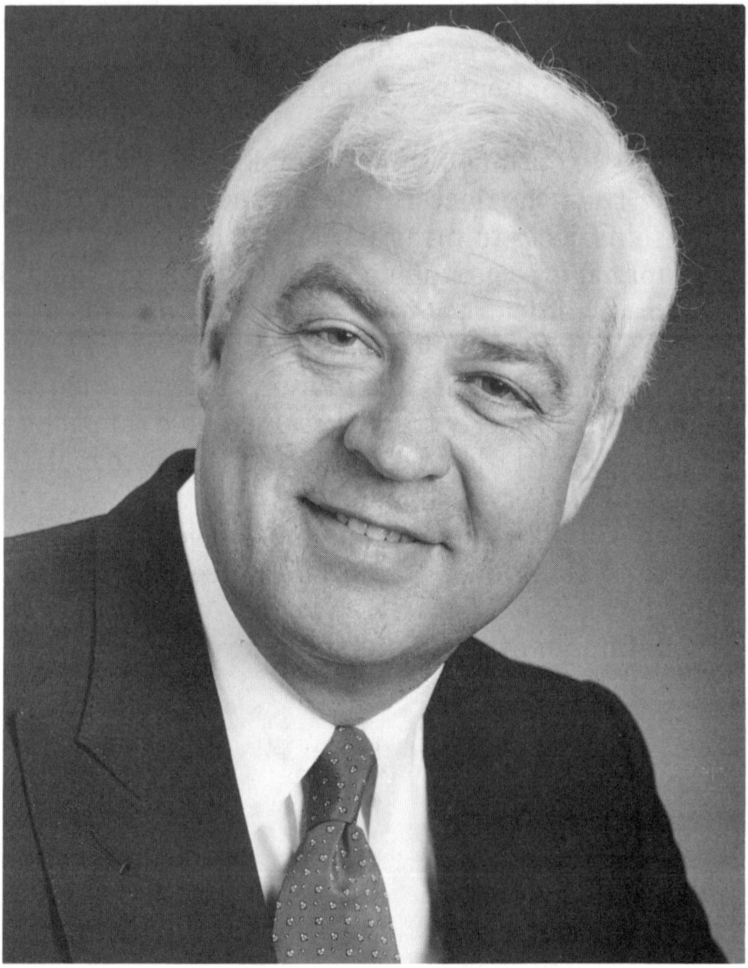

John T. Whitney, D.C.

JOHN WHITNEY, D.C.

AUDIO-VISUAL MANAGEMENT CORPORATION

I believe the healing process begins at the moment the patient telephones the doctor's office for an appointment. From this first contact, the patient must feel he/she has made the right decision to visit an office that projects an expectation of fulfilling his/her personal needs.

To make this simple formula for success work in your office requires every staff member - from receptionist to CA - to fully understand the laws of human conviction . . . plus a willingness to apply these positive attitudes on a daily basis.

These concepts - gained from experience in practice and from observation of other "management plans" - are unique. They are the heart of the AUDIO-VISUAL MANAGEMENT CORPORATION (AVMC), a Practice Management model I have developed.

The video technology used in our training format increases your potential to functionally incorporate the principles of modern psychology which, in turn, will broaden the base of your practice.

You will learn to establish a positive atmosphere in your office. AVMC teaches, trains and puts in place the tools you need to provide a total health package . . . the steps which lead to ultimate success in chiropractic.

AUDIO-VISUAL MANAGEMENT CORPORATION
44 MacDonnell Street, Guelph, Ontario NIH 2Z3
(519) 822-4205

NOTES / GOALS:

CHAPTER 7
What You Get Is What You "See"

John Whitney, D.C.

Close your eyes for a minute.

Imagine yourself an unbiased, intelligent, non-judgemental observer. Your assignment is to size up a particular individual - yourself.

Observe this person arising in the morning and making their way through the day. . . analyze the thoughts, actions, inner dialogue and decisions. How does this person look? sound? communicate? Do you find this to be an attractive, amiable, honest, warm, dedicated, caring, enthusiastic, tactful, disciplined individual? One who possesses a powerful belief system, one who generates faith, and one who has confidence in what they do in the office, and in chiropractic?

A sobering scenario, isn't it?

MATCHING BEHAVIOUR TO GOALS

Kenneth Blanchard wrote in his "One Minute Manager": "Look at your goals; look at your performance". . . do they match? Does your behaviour match your goals?

Your "behaviour" is a direct reflection of what is going on inside your head. Your behaviour is the physical manifestation of the thoughts that you constantly think – your "dominant thought" as Dennis Waitley has aptly termed it.

It has been determined in repeated experimentation in non-verbal communication that no matter how we try, we cannot hide what we really feel. No matter how clever your phrasing and how contrived your procedures, people will get the true message eventually.

"Procedures" then are not enough to make you a successful chiropractor.

Surely, we require good, honest and efficient procedures to operate our offices, but to simply parrot "selling phrases" and design a clever Report-of-Findings while smiling constantly like a TV pitchman will not make it in chiropractic.

True, some rituals are often necessary in the proper execution of your duties, but they will not stand alone; not for long.

D.C. BURNOUT IS REAL

Early in my career as a consultant I was surprised and mystified in finding "burnout" among younger chiropractors.

Looking at the surface, these "young lions" had it made! Seemingly, they had good practices, financial security, were well educated . . . but there was a hidden flaw. These were "procedure doctors." A closer scrutiny showed they did all the right things but their practices had no soul, no dedication to a cause, no basic philisophy of practice. Truly, they seemed not to really understand the forces they were working with.

I posed the rhetorical question: "Could Mother Teresa have burnout?" Why not? Could understanding of fundamental principles of how the world works have anything to do with it? I think so.

HOW THE WORLD WORKS

How does the world work? A few teachers have given us direction. Emerson said that "the universe is plastic and fluid and takes our impress." Thoreau: "if one advances *confidently* in the direction of his dreams and endeavors to live the life which he has *imagined*, he will meet with success." Jesus: "if thou would but believe; all things are possible." Charlie Brown: "I have met the enemy, and they is us."

Does this all imply that success in this world is an inside job, a head trip? Does this imply that good luck or genetics or education are insignificant? The answer seems to be yes and no. Our genetics alone, our education alone, our luck alone, may not be sufficient to ensure success, but more importantly, *they need not constrain us!*

Hard work is not always the way to prosperity, but is sometimes necessary. Inner attitude and conviction are major factors in the success process. Observe the creations of the human mind which are readily perceived all around us. See the many things that have been designed and built to enhance your comfort and to make life better for you.

Originally these were just thoughts in someone's mind. A clear image in your mind of what you would like to experience is helpful in contributing to the formation of your personal world. If you cannot clearly image your heart's desire, at least inwardly grasp the ideal in general terms and then leave it up to the creative process to arrange the details.

SOLVE THE POPULAR RIDDLE

In order to solve the riddle of success it must first be defined.

"The progressive realization of a worthy ideal" is the definition offered by Earl Nightengale in his "Greatest Secret": "Worthy" really has no place in the definition because it is a moral judgement, but other than that this seems to describe "success" for most people.

So much has been written on success that it often becomes trite.

All the wise men, prophets, philosophers, sages, industrialists, consultants, analysts, and general all-round "doers" who have written on the subject disagree on many things, but there is one thing on which they all agree. We become what we think about most of the time. That's it! Simple.

The next step, then, is to devise a plan for thinking about the things you want to see in your life.

Caution: this is not the equivalent of thinking about what you don't want to see in your life. "I don't want to see less than 50 patients daily" is not the same message to your reticular activating system as "I want to see at least 50 patients daily"; if you miss this subtle point, you lose. The affirmation should *not* be stated in the negative.

So, the composition of your thoughts is a first critical step. This is often where "positive thinkers" go down the drain. Positive thinking doesn't work. Positive thinking is a step only.

If you sit in your office everyday, day after day, thinking wonderful thoughts about your future: co-operative patients, abundant referrals, material success, harmonious family and social life, self-confidence and esteem, you will get results all right. The sheriff will be at your door! "Faith without works is dead."

ACTION - A KEY INGREDIENT

Action is now needed. What sort of action?

It is true that those who operate from a genuine, altruistic vantage seem to do well no matter what. You've seen them. Dr. James Parker calls them "naturally right." They are wonderful people to be around, they have an aura and a warmth that is a joy to observe. They don't have eyeballs, they have two glowing coals! Lovely people. How many do you see? Not a lot, unfortunately. Most of us mortals have to work at it and that's where "right action" comes in. That I ask you to "fake it 'til you make it" does not imply that hypocrisy is being suggested. Simply look, feel, act, radiate, dress, talk, move, react, like the person you really want to be. "Be who you want to be."

If you do this consistently, regularly, with the discipline demanded by the task, you will be transformed as if by magic. Mind you, the proper thought must precede the action or you will develop into a hollow automaton just as surely as the proper technique will ensure positive results.

Office procedure, then, does have a very specific role to play - in the correct sequence, with the correct emphasis.

It is unfortunate, but true, that most chiropractors still seem to cling to the idea that procedure alone is "where it's at." Please abandon this idea if it still rattles through the catacombs of your mind. Please. This erroneous concept has been the eventual downfall of many naive practitioners. The pattern is familiar; the practitioner takes a course in practice building and either does not hear or chooses to neglect the introductory remarks of the speaker who advises correct thinking and mind set prior to the employment of some specific office procedure.

The chiropractor goes home and remembers little about thinking and feeling but has taken voluminous notes on office procedure and clever phrasing which he hastens to employ in the office. The practice takes off. Outwardly the scenario appears to be very constructive and worthwhile.

After a few years of this, the doctor feels empty, fatigued, lethargic. "It's not fun anymore," you'll hear them say. Burnout has begun. It's a bad feeling.

I well remember sitting beside a chiropractor at a Parker seminar. It was Thursday, the day Dr. Parker gives you the unvarnished truth of practice. "When are we going to be done with this crap and get to the good stuff (procedure)," he said to me. I was so astonished and annoyed that I held my tongue. Anything I would say at that point would have fallen on deaf ears. This type of thinking is not typical in chiropractic, but common I suspect.

THE MECHANICS OF THINKING "RIGHT"

Most of us do have to learn techniques and procedure to complement right thinking, not *replace* it.

Right thinking plus right action leads to rewarding results, an unbeatable combination. It's called "success."

It would appear our attitude has a great deal to do with our progressive realization of an ideal: "Success." Can attitude be defined?

I offer this definition: attitude is the sum total of what we think, feel, and act. No more no less.

Most people agree that the last word in this trio, "act," is the final gauge by which people judge us. How we conduct ourselves ("act") will ultimately be responsible for the results we get in our lives. How we act is the result of how we think.

How does one change one's thinking? Can one change one's thinking? Absolutely. Is it simple? Yes, (but not easy).

The fact is, we alone are responsible for the thoughts we think. We choose them. It's called "free will."

You don't have to exercise your free will if you choose not to. You don't have to reason on various impressions that reach your mind via your senses - sight, sound, touch, smell, taste. "Things go better with Coke" is an impression (advertising) from the outside world. You can accept it (set free will aside); or your can reject it by thinking about it rationally since you may be aware that many consider the ingredients of Coke to be toxic.

RESULTS = THOUGHTS

The results you get in your practice are due to the thoughts you think; your thoughts about what chiropractic is and what it is capable of doing.

Have you ever noticed your zeal and enthusiasm upon mastering a new technique? No challenge is too great. Bring on the halt, the blind and the lame! Have you ever noticed the empty feeling and marginal results that the same technique brings after it has fallen from your favour?

What is going on? What force(s) are at work in these common occurrences?

William Osler, acclaimed as the father of modern medicine, once said: "Use the new (treatment) quickly before it loses its effectiveness." He appears to have understood that what goes on in the doctor's head will have a significant impact on the results he gets.

The question remains: how do we *change* our thinking?

Edward de Bono, the British scholar, has devised a whole system to teach people to think; he calls it lateral thinking. The system is presently being used in countries all over the world. Karl Albrecht of California goes into considerable detail in his how-to-think book, "Brain Power," on how people can master the "Art of Clear Thinking," as Rudolph Flesch called his book many years ago.

The limitations of space do not allow me to explore the minute details of how one thinks, but I assure you that all those who teach "thinking" agree with the early assertion, "We become what we think about, most of the time." So, let's simplify things: What are you thinking about? What occupies your conscious thought most of the time? Fear? Anxiety over "making it?" Worry about the future? Fear, anxiety, and worry are not fertile grounds for successful life experiences.

What is your "dominant thought?" Do you generally have an attitude of positive expectancy? Do you feel worthy of success? Do you have well-established goals and *fully expect* to realize them?

With this background information, let's get an image to work with.

Our minds need images. We cannot learn much by dealing with abstractions it seems. I offer you a working hypothesis. This theoretical construct will give you a working plan for thinking rationally and for helping you to understand the depth and importance of ATTITUDE.

William James said, "The greatest discovery of my generation is that human beings can alter their lives by altering their ATTITUDES of mind."

WHAT ATTITUDE IS

Attitude is the composite of your THOUGHTS, FEELINGS and ACTIONS. Your ATTITUDE is everything about you. It is not just your thoughts. It is not just your feelings. It is not just your actions. It is the composite of all three and, as already mentioned, it affects your entire life.

To properly understand what attitude is, it becomes necessary to study three basic parts of your personality and how they work:

Part One . . . . THOUGHTS
Part Two . . . . FEELINGS
Part Three . . . . ACTIONS

As you seriously study and understand the three parts of your personality and the LAWS governing them, you will become aware what a mighty energy is set in motion with each mental ATTITUDE.

The part of your personality you can see is, of course, your BODY and this part is the part that moves into ACTION. This represents one of the ingredients of your ATTITUDE.

The other two parts of your personality are the ones you cannot see. These are the CONSCIOUS MIND and the

SUB-CONSCIOUS MIND. The CONSCIOUS MIND deals with THOUGHTS and the SUB-CONSCIOUS MIND with FEELINGS. They are the other two ingredients that make up your ATTITUDE.

Whatever we are *thinking* (FCB) will be reflected in how we are *feeling*; our feelings are always reflected in our *actions*. This is the basic, fundamental process in all human behaviour.

This is the process that goes on in your life and in your practice. This process is the reason why it is critical to be very selective in your thinking and especially in your "self-talk."

Understanding this process will – once and for all – help you to abandon the idea that successful chiropractic practice results from simply employing some nifty procedures (e.g. the perfect consultation, a dazzling report of findings, clever phrasing).

Using procedure as a basis for excellence in your office is like a man climbing a tree to get to the moon: rapid progress is made at first but the shortcomings of the project become apparent in the uppermost branches.

If you merely use "good office procedure" without developing a complete understanding of thinking (FCB) and feeling, you are employing only one-third of the three necessary ingredients. The practice will "fail" by failing to thrive or by leading to boredom, depression and ennui. Burnout.

Remember Mother Teresa; how do you think she feels about her work? Would "enthusiastic" be too mild a term? Do you suppose she may have a powerful FCB in the merit of her work?

We, you and me, will get where we want to go not by reaching out – but by reaching in. (Seek ye first the kingdom within).

As mentioned earlier, to bring order and understanding

to your mind, you must have an image to work with.

Since your mind is the unseen part of your personality, you must engage your imagination to build this image. This can be accomplished with a simple model (Fig. 1) that will help you understand the ingredients of attitude or personality.

FACTORS OF THE PERSONALITY

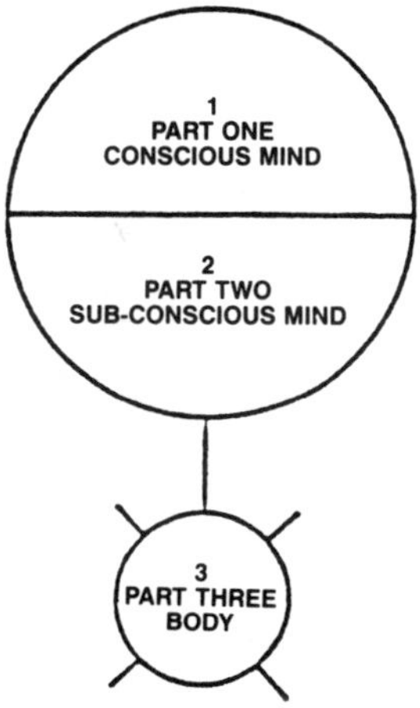

Fig. 1

This simple diagram is used as a working hypothesis to graphically illustrate three basic parts of the human personality.

The "Stickman," like some other ideas presented, is extremely simple. Do not let its simplicity deceive you. This working model reveals a wonderful world of power, possibility and promise. It is a theoretical construct.

This entire construct is built on the premise that you have a power within you that is far superior to any conditions or circumstances around you. With FREE WILL your thoughts direct this power for whatever results you choose in this lifetime. D.D. Palmer was an advocate of this idea.

CONSCIOUS MIND RECEPTORS

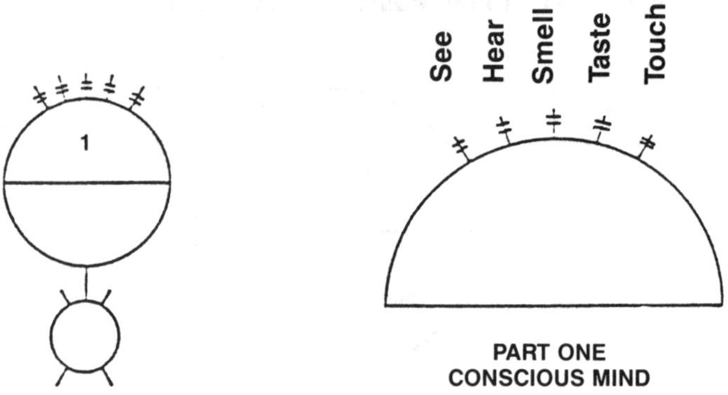

Fig. 2

This is the part of you that thinks - reasons; your free will lies here (Fig. 2). The conscious mind can accept or reject any idea. No person or circumstances can cause you to think about thoughts or ideas you do not choose. The "thoughts" you choose, eventually determine the results in your life. All pain, pleasure and limitation are either originated in the conscious mind or accepted uncritically from an outside source.

As you accept a thought, it is impressed upon the second part of your personality.

"As thou believeth, so shall it be done unto you."

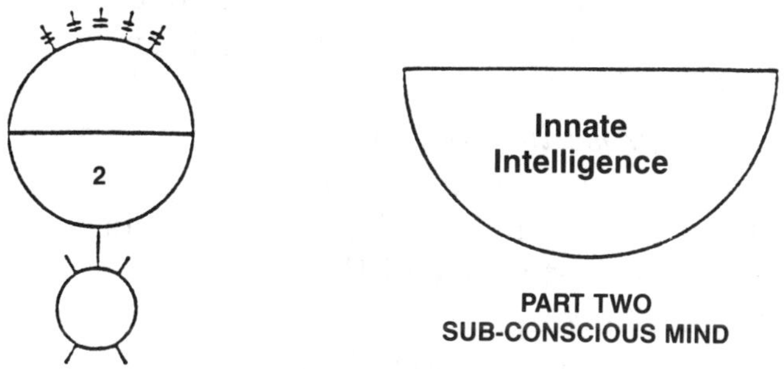

Fig. 3

This part of you is certainly the most magnificent (Fig. 3). It is your power center. It functions in every cell of your body. Every thought your conscious mind chooses to accept, this part must accept . . . it has no ability to reject. This is your "innate intelligence."

This part of you operates in an absolute manner. It expresses itself through you in feelings and action. Any thought you consciously choose to impress upon the subconscious over and over, becomes fixed in this part of your personality. Fixed ideas (concepts) will then continue to express themselves without any conscious assistance, until they are replaced. (Fixed ideas are more commonly referred to as habits). This is the God-like part of you, referred to as Spirit. It knows no limits, save those you consciously choose.

Read: "Power of the Sub-Conscious,"
by Dr. Joseph Murphy
"Three Magic Words," by U.S. Anderson

You and I have self-imposed limitations; they are called "Concepts" or "Ideas." The only truth or reality they have, we give them. We give them this reality because at the time of acceptance we believed them to be "true"; they appeared to our conscious mind and we accepted them on blind faith or after we reasoned upon them. One could say: "that was our attitude at the time." As we have seen, this attitude describes and *proscribes* our activity and achievement.

If we want to change any of our present fixed ideas (concepts), we must simply replace them with other ideas. This is accomplished in one of three ways:

1) Rational Thinking: (very rare) – we may be moved by logical argument based on sound reasoning and principle. Most of us think that this is how *we* think. I wish it were true.

2) Fascination: (very common) – this is the process by which most of us accept anything. You probably don't believe me, but it's true. (The people who sell us soap, booze, tobacco, cars, know that it's true).

3) Repetition: (especially while in a relaxed state) – this is an effective mechanism but can require considerable personal discipline. Repetition is the basis of "brainwashing" and will work for anyone who is reasonably receptive and desirous of change. This mechanism is also used in advertising ("how do you spell relief")?

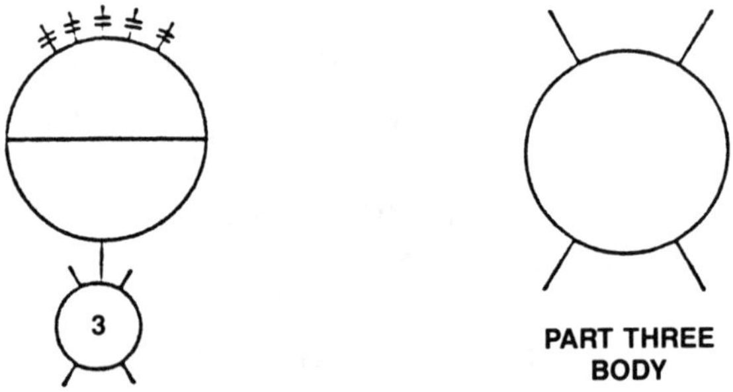

Fig. 4

Although this is the most obvious part of you, it is the smallest part (Fig. 4). The body is the physical representation of you . . . the material medium, it is merely the instrument of the mind, or the house you live in. The thoughts or images that are chosen, impressed upon the sub-conscious (which is in every cell of your body), must move your body into action. The actions in which you are involved determine your results.

ATTITUDE AND RESULTS

Either choose your thoughts or accept them from an outside source. These thoughts develop into images or ideas in your conscious mind. You then impress the images upon your sub-conscious mind, which cause feelings or vibrations. The feelings or vibrations cause actions and the actions cause the results you are getting in your life (Fig. 5).

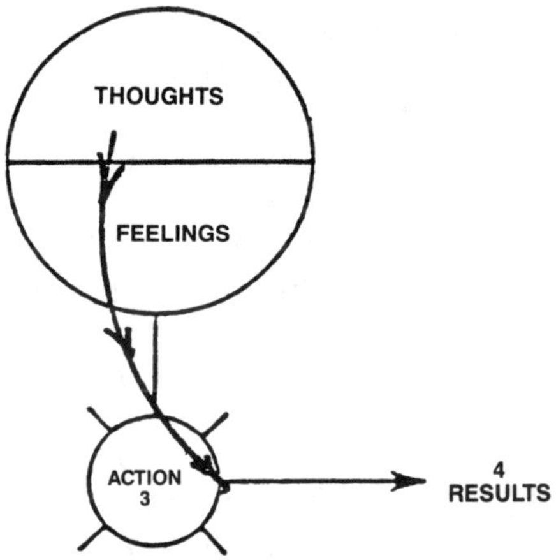

Fig. 5

Your ATTITUDE is the composite of your THOUGHTS, FEELINGS and ACTIONS. The only way to improve the results you are getting in your life is to take full responsibility for your RESULTS. Only then will you be able to improve your ATTITUDE.

The results in your practice (life) are not due to: your mother-in-law, the school you graduated from, your astrological sign, good luck, bad luck, your sister Edna, your adjusting table, your lazy C.A., your Karma, or your haircut - just your attitude.

Summary:

If we are not pleased with the results in our lives, we must merely backtrack.

Think + Feel + Act = Results in life

This leads us to acting differently; but we said action alone ("procedure") is not the answer, so let's backtrack a little more to "feel." What governs the way we feel?

Think + Feel + Act = Results in life

The way you and I "feel" results from the thoughts that we think; especially those thoughts we *frequently* think.

Think + Feel + Act = Results in life

I'm afraid there is no escape. Logic, pure syllogism leads us to the conclusion that if you and I are to change the results in our lives, we must change our thinking.

Think + Feel + Act = Results in life

Success in operating a chiropractic office is no different from success in operating your life or General Motors. Principles are principles; learn them and use them – and never lose sight of one fundamental and inescapable truth. . . .

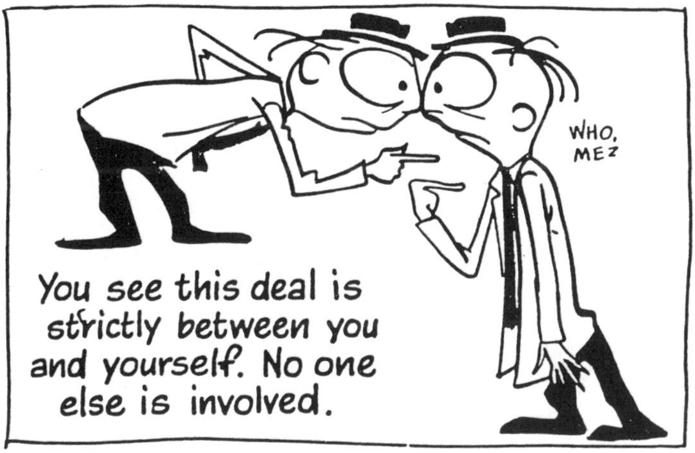

"YOU ARE THE ONLY
PROBLEM
YOU WILL EVER HAVE
AND
YOU ARE THE ONLY
SOLUTION"

**DR. WHITNEY'S
SEVEN STEPS TO CHIROPRACTIC SUCCESS**

1) Clear image of the goal
2) Positive expectancy
3) Persistence
4) Energy
5) Personal integrity
6) Double win strategy
7) Be the solution to your problem.

NOTES / GOALS:

NOTES / GOALS:

NOTES / GOALS:

NOTES / GOALS:

NOTES / GOALS: